A FEAST OF INFORMATION—
for people who love to eat but need to know
the calorie count of their meals.

THE BARBARA KRAUS 1982 CALORIE
GUIDE TO BRAND NAMES & BASIC FOODS
lists thousands of basic and ready-to-eat foods
from appetizers to desserts—carry it to the
supermarket, to the restaurant, to the beach, to
the coffee cart, and on trips.

Flip through these fact-filled pages. Mix, match,
and keep track of calories as they add up. But
remember, strawberry shortcake is fattening any
way you slice it!

The Barbara Kraus 1982 Calorie Guide to Brand Names and Basic Foods

SIGNET Books for Your Reference Shelf

☐ **THE LOS ANGELES TIMES NATURAL FOOD COOKBOOK by Jeanne Voltz, Food Editor, Women's Day Magazine.** Discover the joys of cooking and eating naturally with this book of over 600 savory, simple-to-follow recipes. Whether you are concerned with taste or nutrition, these delicious and healthy recipes—high in fiber content—will delight everyone from the gourmet chef to the dedicated dieter. (#E9038—$2.95)

☐ **CALORIES AND CARBOHYDRATES by Barbara Kraus: Foreword by Edward B. Greenspan, M.D.** Revised edition. This dictionary contains 8,000 brand names and basic foods with their caloric and carbohydrate counts. Recommended by doctors, nutritionists, and family food planners as an indispensable aid to those who must be concerned with what they eat, it will become the most important diet reference source you will ever own. (#E9589—$2.95)

☐ **THE JEWISH LOW-CHOLESTEROL COOKBOOK by Roberta Leviton, with an introduction by Rabbi Meyer J. Strassfeld.** This modern, health-conscious cookbook offers over 200 taste-tempting recipes from around the world to help you cut your cholesterol and lose weight without sacrificing any of those traditional favorites. (#E8623—$2.50)

☐ **LIVING SALT FREE ... AND EASY by Anna Houston Thorburn with Phyllis Turner.** The first specific guide to medically approved low sodium foods for those who want to live to eat as well as eat to live. Includes a sizable collection of recipes that tastes too good to be diet food! (#W7120—$1.50)

☐ **GOURMET COOKING BY THE CLOCK by William and Chesbrough Rayner.** Here at last are full instructions to one of the fine points of cooking ... the art of perfect timing. These are easy-to-follow recipes for everything from appetizers to desserts with each step of preparation and cooking timed by the clock. (#J9044—$1.95)

Buy them at your local bookstore or use this convenient coupon for ordering.
THE NEW AMERICAN LIBRARY, INC.,
P.O. Box 999, Bergenfield, New Jersey 07621
Please send me the books I have checked above. I am enclosing $_____
(please add $1.00 to this order to cover postage and handling). Send check or money order—no cash or C.O.D.'s. Prices and numbers are subject to change without notice.

Name_____

Address_____

City _____ State _____ Zip Code _____

Allow 4-6 weeks for delivery.
This offer is subject to withdrawal without notice.

The Barbara Kraus 1982 Calorie Guide to Brand Names and Basic Foods

A SIGNET BOOK
NEW AMERICAN LIBRARY
TIMES MIRROR

NAL BOOKS ARE AVAILABLE AT QUANTITY DISCOUNTS
WHEN USED TO PROMOTE PRODUCTS OR SERVICES. FOR
INFORMATION PLEASE WRITE TO PREMIUM MARKETING DIVISION,
THE NEW AMERICAN LIBRARY, INC., 1633 BROADWAY,
NEW YORK, NEW YORK 10019.

Copyright © 1971, 1973, 1975, 1976, 1977 by Barbara Kraus.
© 1978 by John R. Fernbach, Esq. and Murray Cohen,
Co-Executors to the Estate of Barbara Kraus.
Copyright © 1979, 1980, 1981 by The New American Library, Inc.

All rights reserved.

Excerpted from *Dictionary of Calories and Carbohydrates*

SIGNET TRADEMARK REG. U.S. PAT. OFF. AND FOREIGN COUNTRIES
REGISTERED TRADEMARK—MARCA REGISTRADA
HECHO EN CHICAGO, U.S.A.

SIGNET, SIGNET CLASSICS, MENTOR, PLUME, MERIDIAN AND NAL
BOOKS are published by The New American Library, Inc.,
1633 Broadway, New York, New York 10019

FIRST PRINTING, JANUARY, 1982

1 2 3 4 5 6 7 8 9

PRINTED IN THE UNITED STATES OF AMERICA

For Phil, Maryann, Anthony,
Christine and Denise Mandola

Foreword

The composition of the foods we eat is not static: it changes from time to time. In the case of *brand-name* products, manufacturers alter their recipes to reflect the availability of ingredients, advances in technology, or improvements in formulae. Each year new products appear on the market and some old ones are discontinued.

On the other hand, information on *basic foods* such as meats, vegetables, and fruits may also change as a result of the development of better analytical methods, different growing conditions, or new marketing practices. These changes, however, are usually relatively small as compared with those in manufactured products.

Some differences may be found between the values in this book and those appearing on the product labels. This is usually due to the fact that the Food and Drug Administration permits manufacturers to round the figures reported on labels. The data in this book are reported as calculated without rounding. If large differences between the two sets of values are noted, they may be due to changes in product formulae, and in those cases the label data should be used.

For all these reasons, a book of calorie or nutritive values of foods must be kept up to date by a periodic reviewing and revision of the data presented.

Therefore, this handy calorie counter will provide each year the most current and accurate estimates available. Generous use of this little book will help you and your family to select the right foods and the proper number of calories each member requires to gain, lose, or maintain healthy and attractive weight.

Good eating in 1982! For 1983, we'll pick up the new products, drop any has-beens, and make whatever other changes are necessary.

Barbara Kraus

Why This Book?

Some of the data presented here can be found in more detail in my best-selling *Calories and Carbohydrates*, a dictionary of 8,000 brand names and basic foods. Complete as it is, it is meant to be used as a reference book at home or in the office and not to be squeezed into a suit jacket or evening bag—it's just too big.

Therefore, responding to the need for a portable calorie guide, and one which can reflect food changes often, I have written this smaller and handier version. The selection of material and the additional new entries provide readers with pertinent data on thousands of products that they would prepare at home to take to work, eat in a restaurant or luncheonette, nibble on from the coffee cart, take to the beach, buy in the candy store, etcetera.

For the sake of saving space and providing you with a greater selection of products, I had to make certain compromises: whereas in the giant book there are several physical descriptions of a product, here there is but one.

For Beginners Only

The language of dieting is no more difficult to learn than any other new subject; in many respects, it's much easier, particularly if you restrict your education to clearly defined goals.

For you who never before had the need or the interest in a lesson in weight control, I offer the following elementary introduction, applicable to any diet, self-initiated or suggested by your doctor, nutritionist, or dietician.

A Calorie

An analysis of foods in terms of calories is most often the chosen method to describe the relative energy yielded by foods.

A calorie is a shorthand way to summarize the units of energy contained in any foodstuff or alcoholic beverage, similar to the way a thermometer indicates heat. One pound of fat is equal to 3,500 calories. Add this number of calories to those you need to balance your energy requirements and you will gain one pound; subtract it and you will lose a pound.

Other Nutrients

Carbohydrates—which include sugars, starches, and acids—are only one of several chemical compounds in foods that yield calories. Proteins, found mainly in beef, poultry, and fish; fats, found in oils, butter, marbling of meat, poultry skin; and alcohol, found in some beverages, also contribute calories. Except for alcohol, most foods contain at least some of all these nutrients.

The amount of carbohydrates varies from zero in meats and a trace in alcohol to a heavy concentration in sugar, syrups, some fruits, grains, and root vegetables.

As of this date, the most respected nutritional researchers insist that some carbohydrate is necessary every day for maintaining good health. The amount to be included is an individual matter, and in any drastic effort to change your eating patterns, be sure to consult your doctor first.

Now, on how to use this new language.

To begin with, you use this book like a dictionary. If your plan is to cut down on calories, the easiest way to do so is to consult the portable calorie counter and keep an accurate count of your total intake of food and beverages for a period of seven days. If you have not gained or lost weight during that week, divide that number by seven and you'll have your maintenance diet expressed in calories. To lose weight, you must reduce your daily or weekly intake of calories below this maintenance level. (To gain, increase the intake.)

Keeping in mind that you want to stay healthy and eat well-balanced meals (which include the basic food groups: milk or milk products; meat, poultry, or fish; vegetables and fruits; and whole grain or enriched breads or cereals, as well as some fats or oils), you then start to cut down on your portion in order to reduce your intake of calories. There are many imaginative ways to diet without total withdrawal from one's favorite foods.

Once you know and don't have to guess what calories are in your foods, you can relax and enjoy it. It could turn out that dieting isn't so bad after all.

ABBREVIATIONS AND SYMBOLS

* = prepared as package directs[1]
< = less than
& = and
″ = inch
canned = bottles or jars as well as cans
dia. = diameter
fl. = fluid
liq. = liquid
lb. = pound
med. = medium

oz. = ounce
pkg. = package
pt. = pint
qt. = quart
sq. = square
T. = tablespoon
Tr. = trace
tsp. = teaspoon
wt. = weight

Italics or name in parentheses = registered trademark, ®. All data not identified by company or trademark are based on material obtained from the United States Department of Agriculture or Health, Education and Welfare/Food and Agriculture Organization.

EQUIVALENTS

By Weight
1 pound = 16 ounces
1 ounce = 28.35 grams
3.52 ounces = 100 grams

By Volume
1 quart = 4 cups
1 cup = 8 fluid ounces
1 cup = ½ pint
1 cup = 16 tablespoons
2 tablespoons = 1 fluid ounce
1 tablespoon = 3 teaspoons
1 pound butter = 4 sticks or 2 cups

---

[1] If the package directions call for whole or skim milk, the data given here are for whole milk unless otherwise stated.

Food and Description	Measure or Quantity	Calories
A		
ABALONE, canned	4 oz.	91
AC'CENT	¼ tsp.	3
ALEXANDER COCKTAIL MIX		
(Holland House)	1 serving	69
ALLSPICE (French's)	1 tsp.	6
ALMOND:		
In shell	10 nuts	60
Shelled, raw, natural with skins	1 oz.	170
Roasted, dry (Planters)	1 oz.	170
ALMOND EXTRACT:		
(Durkee) pure	1 tsp.	13
(Ehler's)	1 tsp.	12
(Virginia Dare) 34.2% alcohol	1 tsp.	10
ALPHA-BITS, cereal (Post)	1 cup	173
AMARETTO DELIGHT		
COCKTAIL (Mr. Boston)	3 fl. oz.	204
AMARETTO DI SARONNO	1 fl. oz.	82
AMARETTO SOUR COCKTAIL		
(Mr. Boston)	3 fl. oz.	123
A.M. FRUIT DRINK (Mott's)	6 fl. oz.	90
ANCHOVY, PICKLED, canned, flat or rolled, not heavily salted, drained	2-oz. can	79
ANISE EXTRACT:		
(Durkee) imitation	1 tsp.	16
(Virginia Dare) 76% alcohol	1 tsp.	22
ANISE SEED, dried	½ oz.	58
ANISETTE:		
(DeKuyper)	1 fl. oz.	95
(Mr. Boston)	1 fl. oz.	88
APPLE:		
Eaten with skin	2½" dia.	66
Eaten without skin	2½" dia.	53
Canned (Comstock):		
Rings, drained	1 ring	30
Sliced	⅛ of 21-oz. can	45
Dried:		
(Del Monte)	1 cup	151
(Sun-Maid)	2-oz. serving	150
Frozen, sweetened	10-oz. pkg.	264
APPLE BROWN BETTY	1 cup	325
APPLE BUTTER (Smucker's) cider	1 T.	38

1

Food and Description	Measure or Quantity	Calories
APPLE-CHERRY JUICE, *Musselman's*	8 fl. oz.	110
APPLE CIDER:		
Canned (Mott's) sweet	½ cup	59
*Mix, *Country Time*	8 fl. oz.	98
APPLE-CRANBERRY DRINK (Hi-C):		
Canned	6 fl. oz.	90
*Mix	6 fl. oz.	72
APPLE-CRANBERRY JUICE (Lincoln)	6 fl. oz.	104
APPLE DRINK:		
Canned:		
(Ann Page)	6 fl. oz.	80
(Hi-C)	6 fl. oz.	92
*Mix (Hi-C)	6 fl. oz.	72
APPLE DUMPLINGS, frozen (Pepperidge Farm)	1 dumpling	280
APPLE, ESCALLOPED, frozen (Stouffer's)	4 oz.	138
APPLE-GRAPE JUICE, canned:		
Musselman's	6 fl. oz.	82
(Red Cheek)	6 fl. oz.	69
APPLE JACKS, cereal (Kellogg's)	1 cup	110
APPLE JELLY:		
Sweetened (Smucker's)	1 T.	67
Dietetic:		
(Dia-Mel) old fashioned	1 T.	6
(Diet Delight)	1 T.	14
(Featherweight)	1 T.	16
(Featherweight) artificially sweetened	1 T.	6
(Slenderella) imitation	1 T.	24
(Tillie Lewis) *Tasti-Diet*	1 T.	11
APPLE JUICE:		
Canned:		
(Ann Page)	½ cup	79
(Lincoln)	6 fl. oz.	96
(Minute Maid)	6 fl. oz.	100
(Mott's)	6 fl. oz.	80
Musselman's	6 fl. oz.	80
(Red Cheek)	6 fl. oz.	83
(Seneca Foods) regular or 100% natural, Vitamin C added	6 fl. oz.	90
Chilled (Minute Maid)	6 fl. oz.	100

Food and Description	Measure or Quantity	Calories
*Frozen:		
(Minute Maid)	6 fl. oz.	100
(Seneca Foods) Vitamin C added	6 fl. oz.	90
(Seneca Foods) natural style, Vitamin C added	6 fl. oz.	84
APPLE PIE (See PIE, Apple)		
APPLE SAUCE:		
Regular:		
(Del Monte)	1 cup	193
(Mott's) natural	½ cup	115
(Mott's) with ground cranberries	4-oz. serving	110
Musselman's	½ cup	96
(Stokely-Van Camp)	½ cup	90
Dietetic:		
(Diet Delight)	½ cup	54
(Featherweight)	½ cup	50
(Mott's) natural	4-oz. serving	50
Musselman's, natural	½ cup	50
(Seneca Foods) 100% natural	½ cup	50
(S&W) *Nutradiet*	½ cup	55
(Tillie Lewis) *Tasti-Diet*	½ cup	61
APPLE SPREAD (Smucker's) low sugar	1 T.	24
APPLE TURNOVER (See TURNOVER)		
APRICOT:		
Fresh, whole	1 apricot	18
Canned, regular		
(Del Monte) whole, peeled	1 cup	208
(Libby's) halves, heavy syrup	1 cup	221
(Stokely-Van Camp)	1 cup	220
Canned, dietetic:		
(Del Monte) *Lite*	½ cup	64
(Diet Delight) syrup pack	½ cup	64
(Diet Delight) water pack	½ cup	35
(Featherweight) juice pack	½ cup	50
(Featherweight) water pack	½ cup	35
(S&W) *Nutradiet*, halves, juice pack	½ cup	50
(S&W) *Nutradiet*, halves, water pack	½ cup	35
(S&W) *Nutradiet*, whole, juice pack	½ cup	40
(Tillie Lewis) *Tasti-Diet*	½ cup	60

Food and Description	Measure or Quantity	Calories
Dried:		
(Del Monte)	½ cup	145
(Sun-Maid)	¼ cup	140
APRICOT LIQUEUR (DeKuyper)	1 fl. oz.	82
APRICOT-PINEAPPLE NECTAR, canned, dietetic (S&W) *Nutradiet*	6-oz. serving	35
APRICOT & PINEAPPLE PRESERVE: Sweetened		
(Smucker's)	1 T.	53
Dietetic:		
(Diet Delight)	1 T.	16
(Featherweight) artificially sweetened	1 T.	6
(S&W) *Nutradiet*	1 T.	12
APRICOT SOUR COCKTAIL (National Distillers-*Duet*) 12% alcohol	2 fl. oz.	48
APRICOT SPREAD, low sugar (Smucker's)	1 T.	24
ARTICHOKE:		
Boiled	12-oz. artichoke	150
Canned (Cara Mia) marinated, drained	6-oz. jar	175
Frozen:		
(Birds Eye) deluxe hearts	⅓ pkg.	34
(Cara Mia)	3-oz. serving	35
ASPARAGUS:		
Boiled	1 spear (½" dia. at base)	3
Canned, regular pack, spears, solids & liq.		
(Del Monte) green or white	1 cup	47
(Green Giant) green	5¼-oz. serving	22
Musselman's	1 cup	40
(Stokely-Van Camp)	1 cup	45
Canned, dietetic, solids & liq.:		
(Diet Delight)	½ cup	18
(Featherweight) cut spears	1 cup	40
(S&W) *Nutradiet*	1 cup	40
Frozen:		
(Birds Eye) cuts	⅓ pkg.	25
(Green Giant) cuts, butter sauce	1 cup	90
(McKenzie)	⅓ pkg.	30
(Seabrook Farms)	⅓ pkg.	30
(Stouffer's) soufflé	⅓ pkg.	118

Food and Description	Measure or Quantity	Calories
ASPARAGUS SOUP (Campbell) cream of	10-oz. serving	100
AUNT JEMIMA (See SYRUP)		
AVOCADO, all varieties	1 fruit	378
AWAKE (Birds Eye)	6 fl. oz.	88
AYDS:		
Butterscotch	1 piece	27
Chocolate, chocolate mint, vanilla	1 piece	26

B

Food and Description	Measure or Quantity	Calories
BAC ONION (Lawry's)	1 tsp.	14
BACON, broiled (Oscar Mayer):		
Regular slice	7-gram slice	41
Thick slice	1 slice	64
BACON BITS:		
(Durkee) imitation	1 tsp.	8
(French's) imitation	1 tsp.	6
(General Mills) *Bac*Os*	1 tsp.	13
(Hormel)	1 tsp.	11
(Oscar Mayer) real	1 tsp.	6
BACON, CANADIAN, unheated:		
(Hormel) sliced	1-oz. serving	50
(Oscar Mayer) 93% fat free	.7-oz. slice	30
(Oscar Mayer) 93% fat free	1-oz. slice	40
BACON, SIMILATED, cooked:		
(Oscar Mayer) *Lean 'N Tasty*:		
Beef	1 slice	39
Pork	1 slice	45
(Swift) *Sizzlean*	1 strip	50
BAGEL (Lender's) garlic, onion or poppyseed	2-oz. bagel	161
BAKING POWDER (Calumet)	1 tsp.	2
BAMBOO SHOOTS:		
Raw, trimmed	¼ lb.	150
Canned, drained:		
(Chun King)	½ of 8½-oz. can	20
(La Choy)	½ of 8½-oz. can	24
BANANA, unpeeled, medium	6.3-oz. banana	101
BANANA EXTRACT (Durkee) imitation	1 tsp.	15
BANANA PIE (See PIE, Banana)		
BARBECUE SEASONING (French's)	1 tsp.	6
BARDOLINO WINE (Antinori)	1 fl. oz.	28

Food and Description	Measure or Quantity	Calories
BARLEY, pearled (Quaker Scotch)	¼ cup	172
BASIL (French's)	1 tsp.	3
BASS:		
Baked, stuffed	3½" x 4½" x 1½"	531
Oven-fried	8¾" x 4½" x ⅝"	392
BAY LEAF (French's)	1 tsp.	5
B & B LIQUEUR	1 fl. oz.	94
B.B.Q. SAUCE & BEEF, frozen (Banquet) sliced	5-oz. cooking bag	126
BEAN, BAKED:		
(USDA):		
With pork & molasses sauce	1 cup	383
With pork & tomato sauce	1 cup	311
Canned:		
(Ann Page) with pork & molasses sauce, Boston style	8 oz.	287
(B&M):		
Pea bean with pork in brown sugar sauce	8 oz.	336
Red kidney bean in brown sugar sauce	8 oz.	360
(Campbell):		
Barbecue	7¾-oz. can	270
Home style	8-oz. can	300
With molasses & brown sugar sauce, old fashioned	8-oz. serving	290
With pork & tomato sauce	8-oz. can	260
(Libby's):		
Deep Brown, with pork & molasses sauce	½ of 14-oz. can	220
Deep Brown, vegetarian in tomato sauce	½ of 14-oz. can	214
(Sultana) with pork & tomato sauce	½ of 16-oz. can	232
(Van Camp) with pork or vegetarian style	1 cup	260
BEAN, BLACK, DRY	1 cup	678
BEAN, BROWN, DRY	1 cup	678
BEAN & FRANKFURTER, canned:		
(Campbell) in tomato and molasses sauce	8-oz. can	370
(Hormel) *Short Orders*, 'n wieners	7½-oz. can	290
BEAN & FRANKFURTER DINNER, frozen:		
(Banquet)	10¾-oz. dinner	691
(Morton)	10¾-oz. dinner	528
(Swanson) TV Brand	11¼-oz. dinner	550

Food and Description	Measure or Quantity	Calories
BEAN, GARBANZO, canned, dietetic (S&W) *Nutradiet*, low sodium	½ cup	105
BEAN, GREEN:		
Boiled, 1½" to 2" pieces, drained	½ cup	17
Canned, regular pack:		
(Comstock) solids & liq.	½ cup	23
(Del Monte) French, drained	½ cup	27
(Green Giant) French or whole, solids & liq.	½ cup	15
(Kounty Kist) French or whole, solids & liq.	½ cup	15
(Libby's) cut, solids & liq.	½ cup	18
(Libby's) French, solids & liq.	½ cup	21
(Stokely-Van Camp) solids & liq.	½ cup	20
Canned, dietetic:		
(Diet Delight) solids & liq.	½ cup	17
(Featherweight) cut or French, solids & liq.	½ cup	25
(S&W) *Nutradiet*, cut, solids & liq., low sodium	½ cup	20
(Tillie Lewis) *Tasti-Diet*, Blue Lake, solids & liq.	½ cup	20
Frozen:		
(Birds Eye):		
Cut	⅓ pkg.	25
With mushroom on onion	⅓ pkg.	32
With toasted almonds	⅓ pkg.	56
(Green Giant):		
With butter sauce	⅓ pkg.	31
With mushroom sauce	⅓ pkg.	38
(McKenzie)	⅓ pkg.	29
(Seabrook Farms)	⅓ pkg.	29
BEAN, GREEN, & MUSHROOM CASSEROLE (Stouffer's)	½ pkg.	143
BEAN, GREEN, PUREE, canned, dietetic (Featherweight)	1 cup	70
BEAN, ITALIAN:		
Canned (Del Monte) drained	½ cup	43
Frozen (McKenzie; Seabrook Farms)	⅓ pkg.	37
BEAN, KIDNEY:		
Canned, regular pack:		
(Ann Page)	¼ of 15½-oz. can	104
(Ann Page) in chili gravy	½ of 15-oz. can	208
(Van Camp) red	1 cup	230

Food and Description	Measure or Quantity	Calories
Canned, dietetic (S&W) *Nutradiet*, low sodium, solids & liq.	½ cup	90
BEAN, LIMA:		
Boiled, drained	½ cup	94
Canned, regular pack		
(Del Monte) drained	½ cup	108
(Libby's) solids & liq.	½ cup	91
(Sultana) butter bean	¼ of 15-oz. can	82
Canned, dietetic (Featherweight) solids & liq.	½ cup	80
Frozen:		
(Birds Eye) baby limas	⅓ pkg.	120
(Birds Eye) Fordhooks	⅓ pkg.	100
(Green Giant) speckled butter beans, Southern recipe	⅓ pkg.	105
(McKenzie) baby limas	⅓ pkg.	126
(McKenzie) baby butter bean	⅓ pkg.	139
(Seabrook Farms) baby limas	⅓ pkg.	126
(Seabrook Farms) baby butter bean	⅓ pkg.	139
(Seabrook Farms) Fordhooks	⅓ pkg.	98
BEAN, RED MEXICAN, canned (Green Giant)	¼ of 15½-oz. can	97
BEAN, REFRIED, canned:		
Old El Paso	½ of 8¼-oz. can	103
(Ortega) lightly spicy or true bean	½ cup	170
BEAN SALAD, canned:		
(Green Giant)	4½-oz. serving	92
(Nalley's)	4½-oz. serving	155
BEAN SOUP:		
*(Ann Page) condensed, with bacon	1 cup	141
(Campbell):		
Chunky, with ham	11-oz. can	300
*Condensed, with bacon	11-oz. serving	190
(Crosse & Blackwell) with sherry	13-oz. can	160
BEAN SPROUT:		
Mung, raw	½ lb.	80
Mung, boiled, drained	¼ lb.	32
Soy, raw	½ lb.	104
Soy, boiled, drained	¼ lb.	43
Canned:		
(Chun King) drained	8 oz.	40
(La Choy) drained	1 cup	13

Food and Description	Measure or Quantity	Calories
BEAN, YELLOW OR WAX:		
Boiled, 1" pieces, drained	½ cup	18
Canned, regular pack:		
(Comstock) solids & liq.	½ cup	22
(Del Monte) cut, solids & liq.	½ cup	19
(Libby's) cut, solids & liq.	4 oz.	23
(Stokely-Van Camp) solids & liq.	½ cup	23
Canned, dietetic (Featherweight) cut, solids & liq.	½ cup	25
Frozen (Birds Eye) cut	⅓ pkg.	30
BEEF, choice grade, medium done:		
Brisket, braised:		
Lean & fat	3 oz.	350
Lean only	3 oz.	189
Chuck, pot roast:		
Lean & fat	3 oz.	278
Lean only	3 oz.	182
Fat, separable, cooked	1 oz.	207
Filet Mignon, See Steak, sirloin, lean		
Flank, braised, 100% lean	3 oz.	167
Ground:		
Regular, raw	½ cup	203
Regular, broiled	3 oz.	243
Lean, broiled	3 oz.	186
Rib:		
Roasted, lean & fat	3 oz.	374
Lean only	3 oz.	205
Round:		
Broiled, lean & fat	3 oz.	222
Lean only	3 oz.	161
Rump:		
Roasted, lean & fat	3 oz.	295
Lean only	3 oz.	177
Steak, club, broiled:		
One 8-oz. steak (weighed without bone before cooking) will give you:		
Lean & fat	5.9 oz.	754
Lean only	3.4 oz.	234
Steak, porterhouse, broiled:		
One 16-oz. steak (weighed with bone before cooking) will give you:		
Lean & fat	10.2 oz.	1339

Food and Description	Measure or Quantity	Calories
Lean only	5.9 oz.	372
Steak, ribeye, broiled:		
One 10-oz. steak (weighed without bone before cooking) will give you:		
Lean & fat	7.3 oz.	911
Lean only	3.8 oz.	258
Steak, sirloin, double-bone, broiled:		
One 16-oz. steak (weighed with bone before cooking) will give you:		
Lean & fat	8.9 oz.	1028
Lean only	5.9 oz.	359
One 12-oz. steak (weighed with bone before cooking) will give you:		
Lean & fat	6.6 oz.	767
Lean only	4.4 oz.	268
Steak, T-bone, broiled:		
One 16-oz. steak (weighed with bone before cooking) will give you:		
Lean & fat	9.8 oz.	1315
Lean only	5.5 oz.	348
BEEFAMATO COCKTAIL (Mott's)	6 fl. oz.	70
BEEF BOUILLON, *MBT*	1 packet	14
BEEF, CHIPPED:		
Cooked, home recipe	½ cup	188
Frozen:		
(Banquet) creamed	5 oz.	124
(Stouffer's) creamed	5½ oz.	231
BEEF DINNER or ENTREE, frozen:		
(Banquet)	11-oz. dinner	312
(Banquet) chopped	11-oz. dinner	443
(Morton)	10-oz. dinner	261
(Morton) *Country Table*, sliced	14-oz. dinner	512
(Morton) *Steak House*, sirloin strip	9½-oz. dinner	896
(Swanson) *Hungry Man*, chopped	18-oz. dinner	730
(Swanson) *Hungry Man*, sliced	12¼-oz. dinner	330
(Swanson) TV Brand, chopped sirloin	10-oz. dinner	460
(Swanson) 3-course	15-oz. dinner	490

Food and Description	Measure or Quantity	Calories
(Weight Watchers) beefsteak with pepper & mushroom	10-oz. meal	387
(Weight Watchers) sirloin, 3-compartment	16-oz. meal	516
BEEF, DRIED, canned:		
(Hormel) *Short Orders*, creamed	7½-oz. can	160
(Swift)	1-oz. serving	47
BEEF GOULASH (Hormel) *Short Orders*	7½-oz. can	230
BEEF, GROUND, SEASONING MIX:		
*(Durkee)	1 cup	653
*(Durkee) with onion	1 cup	659
(French's)	1⅛-oz. pkg.	100
BEEF HASH, ROAST:		
Canned:		
Mary Kitchen	7½-oz. serving	396
Mary Kitchen, Short Orders	7½-oz. can	370
Frozen (Stouffer's)	½ of 11½-oz. serving	262
BEEF AND NOODLES (Banquet)	2-lb. pkg.	754
BEEF PEPPER ORIENTAL, frozen (Chun King):		
Pouch	6 oz.	80
Dinner	11 oz.	310
BEEF PIE, frozen:		
(Banquet)	8-oz. pie	409
(Morton)	8-oz. pie	316
(Stouffer's)	10-oz. pie	552
(Swanson)	8-oz. pie	430
(Swanson) *Hungry Man*	16-oz. pie	770
BEEF PUFFS, frozen (Durkee)	1 piece	47
BEEF, SHORT RIBS, frozen (Stouffer's) boneless, with vegetable gravy	½ of 11½-oz. pkg.	347
BEEF SOUP:		
Canned, regular:		
(Campbell):		
Chunky:		
Regular	10¾-oz. can	190
Regular	19-oz. can	340
With noodles	10¾-oz. can	280
*Condensed		
Regular	11-oz. serving	110
Broth	10-oz. serving	30
Broth & barley	11-oz. serving	90
Broth & noodles	10-oz. serving	80
Consomme	10-oz. serving	45

Food and Description	Measure or Quantity	Calories
Mushroom	10-oz. serving	90
Noodle	10-oz. serving	90
(College Inn) broth	1 cup	18
(Swanson) broth	7¼-oz. serving	20
*Canned, dietetic (Dia-Mel) & noodle	8-oz. serving	70
BEEF SOUP MIX:		
*(Lipton) *Cup-a-Soup*, noodle	6 fl. oz.	35
*(Nestlé) *Souptime*, & noodle	6 fl. oz.	30
BEEF STEAK, BREADED, frozen (Hormel)	4-oz. serving	374
BEEF STEW:		
Home recipe, made with lean beef chuck	1 cup	218
Canned, regular pack:		
Dinty Moore	7½-oz. serving	184
Dinty Moore, Short Orders	7½-oz. can	170
(Libby's)	1 cup	233
(Morton House)	⅛ of 24-oz. can	240
(Nalley's)	7½-oz. serving	226
(Swanson)	7½-oz. serving	190
Canned, dietetic (Dia-Mel)	8-oz. can	200
Frozen:		
(Banquet) buffet	2-lb. pkg.	700
(Green Giant) & biscuits, Bake 'n Serve	14-oz. pkg.	368
(Stouffer's)	10-oz. serving	305
BEEF STEW SEASONING MIX:		
*(Durkee)	1 cup	379
(French's)	1 pkg.	150
BEEF STIX (Vienna)	1 oz.	163
BEEF STROGANOFF, frozen (Stouffer's) with parsley noodles	9¾ oz.	390
***BEEF STROGANOFF SEASONING MIX** (Durkee)	1 cup	320
BEER & ALE:		
Regular:		
Black Horse Ale	8 fl. oz.	108
Black Label	8 fl. oz.	93
Budweiser	8 fl. oz.	103
Busch Bavarian	8 fl. oz.	97
Heidelberg	8 fl. oz.	89
Knickerbocker	8 fl. oz.	107
Meister Brau Premium, regular or draft	8 fl. oz.	96
Michelob	8 fl. oz.	110
North Star, regular	8 fl. oz.	110

Food and Description	Measure or Quantity	Calories
Pearl Premium	8 fl. oz.	99
Pfeifer, regular	8 fl. oz.	110
Pfeifer, 3.2 low gravity	8 fl. oz.	95
Red Cap	8 fl. oz.	102
Rheingold	8 fl. oz.	107
Schmidt, 3.2 low gravity	8 fl. oz.	95
Stag	8 fl. oz.	91
Stroh Bohemian, regular	8 fl. oz.	99
Stroh Bohemian, 3.2 low gravity	8 fl. oz.	84
Tuborg, USA	8 fl. oz.	93
Light or low carbohydrate:		
Gablinger's	8 fl. oz.	66
Meister Brau Lite	8 fl. oz.	64
Michelob, light	8 fl. oz.	89
Natural Light	8 fl. oz.	73
Pearl Light	8 fl. oz.	<1
Stroh Light	8 fl. oz.	77
BEER, NEAR:		
Goetz Pale	8 fl. oz.	53
Kingsbury (Heileman)	8 fl. oz.	30
(Metbrew)	8 fl. oz.	49
BEET:		
Boiled, whole	2" dia. beet	16
Boiled, sliced	½ cup	33
Canned, regular pack:		
(Del Monte) pickled, solids & liq.	½ cup	77
(Del Monte) sliced, solids & liq.	½ cup	29
(Greenwood) Harvard, solids & liq.	½ cup	70
(Greenwood) pickled, solids & liq.	½ cup	110
(Greenwood) pickled, with onion, solids & liq.	½ cup	115
(Libby's) Harvard, solids & liq.	½ cup	87
(Stokely-Van Camp) pickled, solids & liq.	½ cup	95
Canned, dietetic:		
(Blue Boy) whole, solids & liq.	½ cup	39
(Comstock) solids & liq.	½ cup	30
(Featherweight) sliced, solids & liq.	½ cup	45

Food and Description	Measure or Quantity	Calories
(S&W) *Nutradiet*, sliced, solids & liq.	½ cup	35
(Tillie Lewis) *Tasti-Diet*, diced, solids & liq.	½ cup	35
BEET PUREE, canned, dietetic (Featherweight)	1 cup	90
BENEDICTINE LIQUEUR (Julius Wile)	1½ fl. oz.	168
BIG H, burger sauce (Hellmann's)	1 T.	71
BIG MAC (See *McDonald's*)		
BIG WHEEL (Hostess)	1 cake	170
BISCUIT DOUGH (Pillsbury):		
Baking Powder, *1969 Brand*	1 biscuit	100
Big Country	1 biscuit	95
Big Country, Good 'N Buttery	1 biscuit	100
Buttermilk:		
Regular	1 biscuit	50
Ballard, Oven Ready	1 biscuit	50
1869 Brand	1 biscuit	100
Extra Lights	1 biscuit	60
Extra rich, *Hungry Jack*	1 biscuit	65
Flaky, *Hungry Jack*	1 biscuit	80
Fluffy, *Hungry Jack*	1 biscuit	100
Butter Tastin, 1869 Brand	1 biscuit	100
Butter Tastin, Hungry Jack	1 biscuit	95
Country style	1 biscuit	50
Dinner	1 biscuit	55
Flaky, *Hungry Jack*	1 biscuit	90
Heat 'N Eat, *1869 Brand*	1 biscuit	100
Oven Ready, Ballard	1 biscuit	50
Prize	1 biscuit	65
BITTERS (Angostura)	1 tsp.	14
BLACKBERRY, fresh, hulled	1 cup	84
BLACKBERRY JELLY:		
Sweetened (Smucker's)	1 T.	53
Dietetic:		
(Featherweight)	1 T.	16
(Slenderella)	1 T.	24
BLACKBERRY LIQUEUR (Bols)	1 fl. oz.	95
BLACKBERRY PRESERVE OR JAM:		
Sweetened (Smucker's)	1 T.	53
Dietetic:		
(Dia-Mel)	1 T.	6
(Diet-Delight)	1 T.	13
(Featherweight)	1 T.	16
(S&W) *Nutradiet*	1 T.	12

Food and Description	Measure or Quantity	Calories
BLACKBERRY SPREAD, low sugar (Smucker's)	1 T.	24
BLACKBERRY WINE (Mogen David)	3 fl. oz.	135
BLACK-EYED PEAS:		
Canned (Sultana) with pork	7½-oz. serving	130
Frozen:		
(Birds Eye)	⅓ pkg.	130
(Green Giant)	⅓ pkg.	106
(McKenzie)	½ pkg.	130
(Seabrook Farms)	⅓ pkg.	130
BLOODY MARY MIX:		
Dry (Bar-Tender's)	1 serving	26
Liquid (Sacramento)	5½-fl.-oz. can	39
BLUEBERRY, fresh, whole	½ cup	45
BLUEBERRY PIE (See PIE, Blueberry)		
BLUEBERRY PRESERVE OR JAM:		
Sweetened (Smucker's)	1 T.	53
Dietetic (Dia-Mel)	1 T.	6
BLUEFISH, broiled	1½" x 3" x ½" piece	199
BODY BUDDIES, cereal (General Mills):		
Brown sugar & honey	1 cup	110
Natural fruit	¾ cup	100
BOLOGNA:		
(Eckrich):		
Beef, garlic, pickled, ring or sliced	1 oz.	95
Thick sliced	1.7-oz. slice	160
(Hormel):		
Beef	1-oz. slice	86
Coarse ground, ring	1-oz. serving	76
Fine ground, ring	1-oz. serving	82
Meat	1-oz. slice	85
(Oscar Mayer):		
Beef	.5-oz. slice	47
Beef	.8-oz. slice	73
Beef	1-oz. slice	90
Beef	1.3-oz. slice	120
Meat	.5-oz. slice	48
Meat	.8-oz. slice	74
Meat	1-oz. slice	91
(Swift)	1-oz. slice	95
(Vienna) beef	1-oz. serving	84

Food and Description	Measure or Quantity	Calories
BOLOGNA & CHEESE (Oscar Mayer)	.8-oz. slice	73
BONITO, canned (Star-Kist):		
Chunk	6½-oz. can	604
Solid	7-oz. can	650
*BOO*BERRY*, cereal (General Mills)	1 cup	110
BORSCHT (Gold's):		
Regular	8-oz. serving	72
Dietetic	8-oz. serving	24
BOSCO (See SYRUP)		
BOWL O'NOODLES (Nestlé), beef or chicken	1½-oz. envelope	160
BOYSENBERRY JELLY:		
Sweetened (Smucker's)	1 T.	53
Dietetic (S&W) *Nutradiet*	1 T.	12
BOYSENBERRY SPREAD, low sugar (Smucker's)	1 T.	24
BRAN, crude	1 oz.	60
BRAN BREAKFAST CEREAL:		
(Crawford's) & dates	⅛ cup	100
(Kellogg's):		
All Bran or Bran Buds	⅓ cup	70
Cracklin' Bran	⅓ cup	120
40% bran flakes	⅔ cup	90
Raisin	¾ cup	120
(Nabisco)	½ cup	70
(Post) 40% bran flakes	⅔ cup	107
(Quaker) *Corn Bran*	⅔ cup	109
(Ralston-Purina):		
Bran Chex	⅔ cup	90
40% bran	¾ cup	100
Honey	⅞ cup	100
Raisin	¾ cup	120
(Shoprite)	⅝ cup	104
(Van Brode)	⅝ cup	104
BRANDY, FLAVORED (Mr. Boston):		
Apricot	1 fl. oz.	94
Blackberry	1 fl. oz.	92
Cherry	1 fl. oz.	87
Coffee	1 fl. oz.	100
Ginger	1 fl. oz.	72
Peach	1 fl. oz.	94
BRAUNSCHWEIGER:		
(Oscar Mayer) chub	1 oz.	98
(Swift) 8-oz. chub	1 oz.	109

Food and Description	Measure or Quantity	Calories
BRAZIL NUT, shelled	4 nuts	114
BREAD:		
American Granary (Arnold)	.9-oz. slice	70
Boston Brown	3" x ¾" slice	101
Cracked wheat (Wonder)	1-oz. slice	75
Crispbread, *Wasa*:		
Mora	3.2-oz. slice	333
Rye, golden	.4-oz. slice	37
Rye, hearty	.5-oz. slice	54
Rye, lite	.3-oz. slice	30
Sesame	.5-oz. slice	50
Sport	.4-oz. slice	43
Date-nut (Thomas')	1.1-oz. slice	93
Date nut roll (Dromedary)	.5-oz. slice	80
Flatbread, Ideal:		
Bran	.2-oz. slice	19
Ultra thin	.1-oz. slice	12
Whole grain	.2-oz. slice	19
French (Pepperidge Farm)	2-oz. slice	150
French (Wonder)	1-oz. slice	75
Glutogen Gluten (Thomas')	.4-oz. slice	30
Hillbilly (Wonder)	1-oz. slice	70
Hollywood	.6-oz. slice	45
Honey bran (Pepperidge Farm)	1 slice	95
Honey, wheat berry (Arnold)	1.2-oz. slice	90
Italian (Pepperidge Farm)	2-oz. slice	150
Naturel (Arnold)	.9-oz. slice	65
Profile (Wonder) dark	.8-oz. slice	75
Protogen Protein (Thomas')	.7-oz. slice	45
Protogen Protein (Thomas')	.9-oz. slice	55
Pumpernickel:		
(Arnold)	1-oz. slice	75
(Levy's)	1-oz. slice	70
(Pepperidge Farm)	1 slice	80
Raisin:		
(Arnold) tea	.9-oz. slice	70
(Sun-Maid)	1-oz. slice	80
(Thomas') cinnamon	.8-oz. slice	60
Roman Meal	1-oz. slice	70
Rye:		
(Arnold) Jewish	1.1-oz. slice	75
(Levy's) real	1-oz. slice	70
(Pepperidge Farm) family	1 slice	85
(Wonder)	1-oz. slice	60
Sour dough, *Di Carlo*	1-oz. slice	70
Wheat:		
Fresh Horizons	1-oz. slice	54

Food and Description	Measure or Quantity	Calories
Home Pride	1-oz. slice	75
(Pepperidge Farm)	1 slice	95
(Wonder)	1-oz. slice	75
Wheatberry, *Home Pride*	1-oz. slice	70
White:		
(Arnold) *Brick Oven*	.8-oz. slice	65
(Arnold) Melba thin	.5-oz. slice	40
(Levy's) no salt added	.9-oz. slice	80
(Pepperidge Farm):		
Large loaf	1 slice	75
Sandwich	1 slice	65
Sliced, 8-oz. loaf	.8-oz. slice	55
Sliced, 1-lb. loaf	.9-oz. slice	75
Sliced, very thin	1 slice	40
Toasting	1 slice	85
(Wonder)	1-oz. slice	75
Whole wheat:		
(Arnold) *Brick Oven*	.8-oz. slice	60
(Arnold) Melba thin	.5-oz. slice	40
(Pepperidge Farm) thin slice	1 slice	70
(Thomas') 100%	.8-oz. slice	56
BREAD, CANNED, brown, plain or raisin (B&M)	1-oz. slice	52
BREAD CRUMBS (Contadina) seasoned	½ cup	228
*BREAD DOUGH, frozen (Rich's):		
French	1/20 of loaf	59
Italian	1/20 of loaf	60
Raisin	1/20 of loaf	66
*BREAD MIX (Pillsbury):		
Applesauce spice	1/12 of loaf	150
Apricot nut	1/12 of loaf	150
Banana	1/12 of loaf	150
Blueberry nut	1/12 of loaf	150
Cherry nut	1/12 of loaf	170
Cranberry	1/12 of loaf	160
Date	1/12 of loaf	160
Nut	1/12 of loaf	170
BREAD PUDDING, with raisins	½ cup	248
BREAKFAST BAR (Carnation):		
Almond crunch	1 piece	210
All other varieties	1 piece	200
BREAKFAST DRINK:		
(Ann Page)	2 tsp.	63
*(Pillsbury)	1 pouch	130
BREAKFAST SQUARES (General Mills) all flavors	1 bar	190

Food and Description	Measure or Quantity	Calories
BREATH MINTS, dietetic (Featherweight) all flavors	1 piece	4
BRIGHT & EARLY	6 fl. oz.	90
BROCCOLI:		
Boiled, whole stalk	1 stalk	47
Boiled, ½" pieces	½ cup	20
Frozen:		
(Birds Eye) in cheese sauce	⅓ pkg.	110
(Birds Eye) in Hollandaise sauce	⅓ pkg.	100
(Green Giant) spears in butter sauce	⅓ pkg.	43
(Green Giant) in cheese sauce, *Bake 'n Serve*	⅓ pkg.	91
(McKenzie) chopped or spears	⅓ pkg.	111
(Mrs. Paul's) in cheese sauce	⅓ pkg.	161
(Seabrook Farms) chopped or spears	⅓ pkg.	30
(Stouffer's) au gratin	⅓ pkg.	111
BROTH & SEASONING:		
(George Washington)	1 packet	5
Maggi	1 T.	22
BRUSSELS SPROUT:		
Boiled	3-4 sprouts	28
Frozen:		
(Birds Eye)	⅓ pkg.	30
(Birds Eye) baby	⅓ pkg.	42
(Green Giant) in butter sauce	⅓ pkg.	53
(Green Giant) halves in cheese sauce	⅓ pkg.	61
(Kounty Kist)	⅓ pkg.	47
(Stouffer's) au gratin	⅓ pkg.	124
BUCKWHEAT, cracked (Pocono)	1 oz.	104
BUC*WHEATS, cereal (General Mills)	1 oz.	110
BULGUR, canned, seasoned	4-oz. serving	206
BURGER KING:		
Apple pie	3-oz. pie	240
Cheeseburger	1 burger	350
Cheeseburger, double meat	1 burger	530
French fries	1 regular order	210
Hamburger	1 burger	290
Hamburger, double meat	1 burger	420
Onion rings	1 regular order	270
Shake, chocolate or vanilla	1 shake	340

Food and Description	Measure or Quantity	Calories
Whaler	1 sandwich	550
Whaler, with cheese	1 sandwich	650
Whopper	1 burger	630
Whopper, with cheese	1 burger	740
Whopper, Jr.	1 burger	370
Whopper, Jr., with cheese	1 burger	420
BURGUNDY WINE:		
(Great Western)	3 fl. oz.	70
(Italian Swiss Colony)	3 fl. oz.	61
(Louis M. Martini)	3 fl. oz.	90
(Taylor)	3 fl. oz.	75
BURGUNDY WINE, SPARKLING:		
(B&G)	3 fl. oz.	69
(Great Western)	3 fl. oz.	82
(Taylor)	3 fl. oz.	78
BURRITOS, frozen (Hormel):		
Beef	1 burrito	220
Cheese	1 burrito	250
Chicken & rice	4-oz. serving	199
Hot chili	1 burrito	210
BUTTER:		
Regular (Breakstone)	1 T.	100
Regular (Meadow Gold)	1 tsp.	35
Whipped (Breakstone)	1 T.	67
BUTTERSCOTCH MORSELS (Nestlé)	1 oz.	150

C

Food and Description	Measure or Quantity	Calories
CABBAGE:		
Canned:		
(Comstock) red, solids & liq.	½ cup	60
(Greenwood's) red, solids & liq.	½ cup	60
Frozen (Green Giant) stuffed	7 oz. serving	209
CABERNET SAUVIGON (Inglenook)	1 fl. oz.	79
CAFE COMFORT, 55 proof	1 fl. oz.	79
CAKE:		
Regular:		
Plain, home recipe, with butter, with boiled white icing	⅑ of 9″ square	401
Angel food, home recipe	1/12 of 8″ cake	108

Food and Description	*Measure or Quantity*	*Calories*
Caramel, home recipe, with caramel icing	1/9 of 9" square	322
Chocolate, home recipe, with chocolate icing, 2-layer	1/12 of 9" cake	365
Coffee (Tastykake) *Koffee Kakes*	1-oz. cake	124
Fruit, home recipe:		
Dark	1/30 of 8" loaf	57
Light, made with butter	1/30 of 8" loaf	58
Pound, home recipe, traditional, made with butter	3½" x 3½" slice	123
Sponge, home recipe	1/12 of 10" cake	196
White, home recipe, made with butter, without icing, 2-layer	1/9 of 9" wide, 3" high cake	353
Yellow, home recipe, made with butter, without icing, 2-layer	1/19 of cake	351
Frozen:		
Apple walnut (Sara Lee)	1/8 of 12½-oz. cake	165
Banana (Sara Lee)	1/8 of 13¾-oz. cake	175
Banana nut (Sara Lee) layer	1/8 of 20-oz. cake	232
Black forest (Sara Lee)	1/8 of 21-oz. cake	203
Carrot (Sara Lee)	1/8 of 12¼-oz. cake	152
Cheesecake:		
(Morton) *Great Little Desserts:*		
Cherry	6½-oz. cake	476
Cream	6½-oz. cake	489
Pineapple	6½-oz. cake	484
Strawberry	6½-oz. cake	491
(Rich's)	1/16 of cake	212
(Sara Lee):		
Blueberry, *For 2*	½ of 11.3-oz. cake	425
Cherry, *For 2*	½ of 11.3-oz. cake	423
Cream cheese	⅓ of 10-oz. cake	281
Cream cheese	1/6 of 17-oz. cake	231
Cream cheese, blueberry	1/6 of 19-oz. cake	233
Cream cheese, cherry	1/6 of 19-oz. cake	225
Cream cheese, French	1/8 of 23½-oz. cake	274
Cream cheese, strawberry	1/6 of 19-oz. cake	223
Cream cheese, strawberry French	1/8 of 26-oz. cake	258
Strawberry, *For 2*	½ of 11.3-oz. cake	420
Chocolate (Sara Lee):		
Regular	1/8 of 13¼-oz. cake	199

Food and Description	Measure or Quantity	Calories
Bavarian	⅛ of 22½-oz. cake	285
German	⅛ of 12¼-oz. cake	173
Layer, 'n Cream	⅛ of 18-oz. cake	215
Coffee (Sara Lee):		
Almond	⅛ of 11¾-oz. cake	165
Almond ring	⅛ of 9½-oz. cake	135
Apple	⅛ of 15-oz. cake	175
Apple, *For 2*	½ of 9-oz. cake	419
Blueberry ring	⅛ of 9¾-oz. cake	134
Butter, *For 2*	½ of 6½-oz. cake	356
Maple crunch ring	⅛ of 9¾-oz. cake	138
Pecan	¼ of 6½-oz. cake	188
Pecan	⅛ of 11¼-oz. cake	163
Raspberry ring	⅛ of 9¾-oz. cake	133
Streusel, butter	⅛ of 11½-oz. cake	164
Streusel, cinnamon	⅛ of 10.9-oz. cake	154
Crumb (see ROLL OR BUN, Crumb)		
Orange (Sara Lee)	⅛ of 13¾-oz. cake	179
Pound (Sara Lee):		
Regular	1/10 of 10¾-oz. cake	125
Banana nut	1/10 of 11-oz. cake	117
Chocolate	1/10 of 10¾-oz. cake	122
Chocolate swirl	1/10 of 11.8-oz. cake	116
Family size	1/15 of 16½-oz. cake	127
Homestyle	1/10 of 9½-oz. cake	114
Raisin	1/10 of 12.9-oz. cake	126
Strawberries 'n cream, layer (Sara Lee)	⅛ of 20½-oz. cake	193
Torte (Sara Lee):		
Apples 'n cream	⅛ of 21-oz. cake	203
Fudge & nut	⅛ of 15¾-oz. cake	200
Walnut, layer (Sara Lee)	⅛ of 18-oz. cake	210
CAKE OR COOKIE ICING (Pillsbury) all flavors	1 T.	70
CAKE ICING:		
Butter pecan (Betty Crocker) *Creamy Deluxe*	1/12 of can	170
Caramel, home recipe	4 oz.	408
Cherry (Betty Crocker) *Creamy Deluxe*	1/12 of can	170
Chocolate:		
(Betty Crocker) *Creamy Deluxe:*		
Regular	1/12 of can	170
Fudge, dark dutch	1/12 of can	160
Milk	1/12 of can	170

Food and Description	Measure or Quantity	Calories
Nut	1/12 of can	170
Sour cream	1/12 of can	170
(Pillsbury) *Frosting Supreme:*		
Fudge	1/12 of can	160
Milk	1/12 of can	160
Sour cream	1/12 of can	160
Cream cheese:		
(Betty Crocker) *Creamy Deluxe*	1/12 of can	160
(Pillsbury) *Frosting Supreme*	1/12 of can	160
Double dutch (Pillsbury) *Frosting Supreme*	1/12 of can	160
Lemon		
(Betty Crocker) *Sunkist, Creamy Deluxe*	1/12 of can	170
(Pillsbury) *Frosting Supreme*	1/12 of can	160
Orange (Betty Crocker) *Creamy Deluxe*	1/12 of can	170
Strawberry (Pillsbury) *Frosting Supreme*	1/12 of can	160
Vanilla:		
(Betty Crocker) *Creamy Deluxe*	1/12 of can	170
(Pillsbury) *Frosting Supreme*	1/12 of can	160
(Pillsbury) *Frosting Supreme,* sour cream	1/12 of can	160
White:		
Home recipe, boiled	4 oz.	358
Home recipe, uncooked	4 oz.	426
(Betty Crocker) *Creamy Deluxe*	1/12 of can	160
*CAKE ICING MIX:		
Regular:		
Banana (Betty Crocker) *Chiquita,* creamy	1/12 of pkg.	170
Butter Brickle (Betty Crocker) creamy	1/12 of pkg.	170
Butter pecan (Betty Crocker) creamy	1/12 of pkg.	170
Caramel (Pillsbury) *Rich 'n Easy*	1/12 of pkg.	140
Cherry (Betty Crocker) creamy	1/12 of pkg.	170
Chocolate:		
Home recipe, fudge	1/2 cup	586
(Betty Crocker) creamy:		
Fudge	1/12 of pkg.	170
Fudge, dark	1/12 of pkg.	170

Food and Description	Measure or Quantity	Calories
Fudge, sour cream	1/12 of pkg.	170
Milk	1/12 of pkg.	170
(Pillsbury) *Rich 'N Easy:*		
Fudge	1/12 of pkg.	150
Milk	1/12 of pkg.	150
Coconut almond (Pillsbury)	1/12 of pkg.	170
Coconut pecan:		
(Betty Crocker) creamy	1/12 of pkg.	140
(Pillsbury)	1/12 of pkg.	150
Cream cheese & nut (Betty Crocker) creamy	1/12 of pkg.	150
Double dutch (Pillsbury) *Rich 'N Easy*	1/12 of pkg.	150
Lemon:		
(Betty Crocker) *Sunkist,* creamy	1/12 of pkg.	170
(Pillsbury) *Rich 'N Easy*	1/12 of pkg.	140
Strawberry (Pillsbury) *Rich 'N Easy*	1/12 of pkg.	140
Vanilla (Pillsbury) *Rich 'N Easy*	1/12 of pkg.	150
White:		
(Betty Crocker) fluffy	1/12 of pkg.	60
(Betty Crocker) sour cream, creamy	1/12 of pkg.	180
(Pillsbury) fluffy	1/12 of pkg.	70
Dietetic (Betty Crocker) *Lite,* chocolate, lemon or vanilla	1/12 of pkg.	100
CAKE MIX:		
Regular:		
Angel Food:		
(Betty Crocker):		
Chocolate	1/12 pkg.	140
One-step	1/12 pkg.	140
Traditional	1/12 pkg.	130
(Duncan Hines)	1/12 pkg.	124
*(Pillsbury)	1/12 of cake	140
Applesauce raisin (Betty Crocker) *Snackin' Cake*	1/9 pkg.	180
*Applesauce spice (Pillsbury) *Pillsbury Plus*	1/12 of cake	250
Banana:		
*(Betty Crocker) *Super Moist*	1/12 of cake	260
*(Pillsbury) *Pillsbury Plus*	1/12 of cake	260
*(Pillsbury) *Streusel Swirl*	1/16 of cake	260

Food and Description	*Measure or Quantity*	*Calories*
Banana nut (Duncan Hines) *Moist & Easy Snack Cake*	1/9 of pkg.	196
Banana walnut (Betty Crocker) *Snackin' Cake*	1/9 pkg.	190
*Butter (Pillsbury):		
Pillsbury Plus	1/12 of cake	240
Streusel Swirl, rich	1/16 of cake	260
**Butter Brickle* (Betty Crocker) *Super Moist*	1/12 of cake	260
*Butter pecan (Betty Crocker) *Super Moist*	1/12 of cake	250
*Butter yellow (Betty Crocker) *Super Moist*	1/12 of cake	230
*Carrot (Betty Crocker) *Super Moist*	1/12 of cake	260
*Carrot 'n Spice (Pillsbury) *Pillsbury Plus*	1/12 of cake	260
*Cheesecake:		
(Jell-O)	1/8 of 8" cake	250
(Royal)	1/8 of cake	230
*Cherry chip (Betty Crocker) *Super Moist*	1/12 of cake	180
Chocolate:		
(Betty Crocker):		
*Pudding	1/6 of cake	230
Snackin' Cake:		
Almond	1/9 pkg.	190
Fudge chip	1/9 pkg.	190
Stir 'N Frost:		
with chocolate frosting	1/6 pkg.	210
Fudge, with vanilla frosting	1/6 pkg.	210
Super Moist:		
*Fudge	1/12 of cake	250
*German	1/12 of cake	260
*Milk	1/12 of cake	250
*Sour Cream	1/12 of cake	260
*(Pillsbury):		
Bundt:		
Fudge nut crown	1/16 of cake	220
Fudge, triple	1/16 of cake	210
Fudge, tunnel of	1/16 of cake	270
Macaroon	1/16 of cake	250
Pillsbury Plus:		
Fudge, dark	1/12 of cake	260
Fudge, marble	1/12 of cake	270

Food and Description	Measure or Quantity	Calories
German	1/12 of cake	250
Mint	1/12 of cake	250
Streusel Swirl:		
Regular	1/16 of cake	260
German	1/16 of cake	260
Coconut pecan (Betty Crocker) *Snackin' Cake*	1/9 of pkg.	190
Coffee cake:		
*(Aunt Jemima)	1/8 of cake	170
*(Pillsbury):		
Apple cinnamon	1/8 of cake	240
Butter pecan	1/8 of cake	310
Cinnamon streusel	1/8 of cake	250
Sour cream	1/8 of cake	270
Devil's food:		
*(Betty Crocker) *Super Moist*	1/12 of cake	250
(Duncan Hines) pudding recipe	1/12 of cake	187
*(Pillsbury):		
Pillsbury Plus	1/12 of cake	250
Streusel Swirl	1/16 of cake	260
Fudge (See Chocolate)		
Golden chocolate chip (Betty Crocker) *Snackin' Cake*	1/9 of pkg.	190
Lemon:		
(Betty Crocker):		
*Chiffon, *Sunkist*	1/12 of cake	190
Pudding	1/8 of cake	230
Stir 'N Frost, with lemon frosting	1/12 of pkg.	220
Super Moist	1/12 of cake	260
(Duncan Hines) pudding recipe	1/12 of pkg.	183
*(Pillsbury):		
Bundt, tunnel of	1/16 of cake	270
Pillsbury Plus	1/12 of cake	260
Streusel Swirl	1/16 of cake	260
*Lemon blueberry (Pillsbury) *Bundt*	1/16 of cake	200
Marble:		
*(Betty Crocker) *Super Moist*	1/12 of cake	270
*(Pillsbury):		
Bundt, supreme, ring	1/16 of cake	250
Streusel Swirl, fudge	1/16 of cake	260

Food and Description	Measure or Quantity	Calories
*Orange (Betty Crocker) Super Moist	1/16 of cake	260
Pound:		
*(Betty Crocker) golden	1/12 of cake	200
*(Dromedary)	3/4" slice	210
*(Pillsbury) *Bundt*	1/16 of cake	230
Spice (Betty Crocker):		
Snackin' Cake, raisin	1/9 of pkg.	180
Super Moist	1/12 of cake	260
Strawberry:		
*(Betty Crocker) *Super Moist*	1/12 of cake	260
*(Pillsbury) *Pillsbury Plus*	1/12 of cake	260
*Upside down (Betty Crocker) pineapple	1/9 of cake	270
White:		
*(Betty Crocker):		
Stir 'N Frost, with chocolate frosting	1/6 of cake	210
Super Moist	1/12 of cake	180
Super Moist, sour cream	1/12 of cake	180
(Duncan Hines)	1/12 of pkg.	185
(Duncan Hines) pudding recipe	1/12 of pkg.	183
*(Pillsbury) *Pillsbury Plus*	1/12 of cake	240
Yellow:		
*(Betty Crocker) *Super Moist*	1/12 of cake	250
(Duncan Hines)	1/12 of pkg.	186
(Duncan Hines) pudding recipe	1/12 of pkg.	186
*(Pillsbury) *Pillsbury Plus*	1/12 of cake	260
*(Swans Down)	1/12 of cake	185
*Dietetic:		
Chocolate:		
(Betty Crocker) *Light Style*, fudge	1/12 of cake	160
(Estee)	1/10 of cake	100
Devil's food (Betty Crocker) *Light Style*	1/12 of cake	160
Lemon:		
(Betty Crocker) *Light Style*	1/12 of cake	160
(Estee)	1/10 of cake	91

Food and Description	Measure or Quantity	Calories
Yellow (Betty Crocker) *Light Style*	1/12 of cake	160
White (Estee)	1/10 of cake	85
(Dia-Mel) All flavors	1/10 of cake	100
CANDY, REGULAR:		
Almond, chocolate covered (Hershey's) *Golden Almond*	1 oz.	163
Almond, Jordan (Banner)	1¼-oz. box	154
Baby Ruth	1.8-oz. piece	260
Breath Saver (Life Savers)	1 piece	7
Bridge Mix (Nabisco)	1 piece	8
Bun Bars (Wayne)	1 oz.	133
Butterfinger	1.6-oz. bar	220
Butterscotch Skimmers (Nabisco)	1 piece	25
Caramel:		
Caramel Flipper (Wayne)	1 oz.	128
Caramel Nip (Pearson)	1 piece	29
Charleston Chew	1½-oz. bar	179
Cherry, chocolate-covered (Nabisco; *Welch's*)	1 piece	66
Chocolate bar:		
Choco-Lite (Nestlé)	.27-oz. bar	40
Choco-Lite (Nestlé)	1-oz. serving	150
Crunch (Nestlé)	1 1/16-oz. bar	158
Milk:		
(Hershey's)	1.2-oz. bar	187
(Hershey's)	4-oz. bar	623
(Nestlé)	.35-oz. bar	53
(Nestlé)	1 1/16-oz. bar	159
Special Dark (Hershey's)	1.05-oz. bar	160
Special Dark (Hershey's)	4-oz. bar	611
Chocolate bar with almonds:		
(Hershey's) milk	.35-oz. bar	55
(Hershey's) milk	1.15-oz. bar	180
(Hershey's) milk	4-oz. bar	625
(Nestlé)	1-oz. serving	150
(Nestlé)	5-oz. bar	750
Chocolate Parfait (Pearson)	1 piece	31
Chuckles	1 oz.	93
Circus Peanuts (Curtiss)	1 piece	19
Clark Bar	1.4-oz. bar	188
Clark Bar	1.65-oz. bar	222
Cluster, peanut, chocolate-covered (Hoffman)	1 cluster	205
Coconut bar, *Welch's*	1 piece	132
Coffee Nip (Pearson)	1 piece	29

Food and Description	Measure or Quantity	Calories
Coffioca (Pearson)	1 piece	31
Crispy Bar (Clark)	1¼-oz. bar	187
Crispy Bar (Clark)	1.4-oz. bar	209
Crows (Mason)	1 piece	11
Dots (Mason)	1 piece	11
Dutch Treat Bar (Clark)	1¹⁄₁₆-oz. bar	160
Dutch Treat Bar (Clark)	1.3-oz. bar	196
Frappe, Welch's	1 piece	132
Fruit Roll (Sahadi):		
Any flavor but strawberry	1 oz.	90
Strawberry	1 oz.	100
Fudge (Nabisco) bar, *Home Style*	1 bar	90
Good & Fruity	1 oz.	106
Good & Plenty	1 oz.	100
Hollywood	1½-oz. bar	185
Jelly bean (Curtiss)	1 piece	12
Jelly rings, *Chuckles*	1 piece	37
Jujubes, *Chuckles*	1 piece	13
Ju Jus:		
Assorted	1 piece	7
Coins or raspberries	1 piece	15
Kisses (Hershey's)	1 piece	27
Kit Kat	.6-oz. bar	80
Kit Kat	1⅛-oz. bar	179
Krackel Bar	.35-oz. bar	52
Krackel Bar	1.2-oz. bar	178
Krackel Bar	4-oz. bar	594
Licorice:		
Licorice Nips (Pearson)	1 piece	29
(Switzer) bars, bites or stix		
Black	1 oz.	94
Cherry or strawberry	1 oz.	98
Chocolate	1 oz.	97
Twist:		
Black (American Licorice Co.)	1 piece	27
Black (Curtiss)	1 piece	27
Red (American Licorice Co.)	1 piece	33
Life Savers, drop	1 piece	10
Life Savers, mint	1 piece	7
Lollipops (Life Savers)	.9-oz. pop	99
Lollipops (Life Savers)	.6-oz. pop	69
Mallo Cup (Boyer)	⁹⁄₁₆-oz. piece	54
Malted milk balls (Brach's)	1 piece	9
Mars Bar (M&M/Mars)	1½-oz. serving	208
Marshmallow (Campfire)	1 oz.	111

Food and Description	Measure or Quantity	Calories
Mary Jane (Miller):		
Small size	1 piece	18
Large size	1 piece	108
Milk Duds (Clark)	¾-oz. box	89
Milk Duds (Clark)	1¼-oz. box	148
Milk Duds (Clark)	1.4-oz. box	166
Milk Shake (Hollywood)	1¼-oz. bar	150
Milky Way (M&M/Mars)	.8-oz. bar	102
Milky Way (M&M/Mars)	1.9-oz. serving	242
Mint or peppermint:		
After dinner (Richardson):		
Jelly center	1 oz.	104
Regular	1 oz.	109
Chocolate-covered		
(Richardson)	1 oz.	106
Cool Mints (Curtiss)	1 piece	21
Jamaica or Liberty Mints		
(Nabisco)	1 piece	24
Mighty Mint (Life Savers)	1 piece	2
Mint Parfait (Pearson)	1 piece	31
Junior mint pattie (Nabisco)	1 piece	10
Peppermint pattie (Nabisco)	1 piece	64
Thin (Nabisco)	1 piece	42
M & M's:		
Peanut	1½ oz.	219
Plain	1½ oz.	202
Mr. Goodbar (Hershey's)	.35-oz. bar	54
Mr. Goodbar (Hershey's)	1½-oz. bar	233
Mr. Goodbar (Hershey's)	4-oz. bar	620
$100,000 Bar (Nestlé)	1¼-oz. bar	175
Orange slices (Curtiss)	1 piece	29
Orange slices (Nabisco)		
Chuckles	1 piece	29
Payday (Hollywood)	1⅓-oz. bar	154
Peanut, chocolate-covered:		
(Brach's)	1 piece	12
(Curtiss)	1 piece	5
(Nabisco)	1 piece	24
Peanut, French burnt (Curtiss)	1 piece	4
Peanut brittle (Planters):		
Jumbo Peanut Block Bar	1 oz.	119
Jumbo Peanut Block Bar	1 piece (4 grams)	61
Peanut butter cup:		
(Boyer)	1.5-oz. pkg.	148
(Reese's)	.6-oz. cup	92
Raisin, chocolate-covered:		
(Curtiss)	1 oz.	120

Food and Description	Measure or Quantity	Calories
(Nabisco)	1 piece	4
Raisinets (BB)	5¢ size	140
Reggie Bar	2-oz. bar	290
Rolo (Hershey's)	1 piece	30
Royals, mint chocolate (M&M/Mars)	1½-oz. serving	202
Sesame crunch (Sahadi)	¾-oz. bar	120
Snickers	1.8-oz. bar	247
Spearmint leaves:		
(Curtiss)	1 piece	32
(Nabisco) Chuckles	1 piece	27
Starburst (M&M/Mars)	1.9-oz. serving	219
Stars, chocolate (Nabisco)	1 piece	15
Sugar Babies (Nabisco)	1 piece	6
Sugar Daddy (Nabisco):		
Caramel sucker	1 piece	121
Nugget	1 piece	27
Sugar Mama (Nabisco)	1 piece	101
Sugar wafer (F & F)	1¼-oz. pkg.	180
Summit, cookie bar (M&M/Mars)	¾-oz. serving	115
Taffy:		
Salt water (Brach's)	1 piece	31
Turkish (Bonomo)	1-oz. bar	108
3 Musketeers	.8-oz. bar	100
3 Musketeers	2-oz. serving	254
Toffee (Kraft) all flavors	1 piece	29
Tootsie Roll:		
Chocolate	.23-oz. midgee	26
Chocolate	¹⁄₁₆-oz. bar	72
Chocolate	¾-oz. bar	86
Chocolate	1-oz. bar	115
Chocolate	1¾-oz. bar	201
Flavored	.6-oz. square	19
Pop, all flavors	.49-oz. pop	55
Pop drop, all flavors	4.7-gram piece	19
Twix, cookie bar (M&M/Mars)	.85-oz. serving	118
Twix, peanut butter cookie bar (M&M/Mars)	.8-oz. serving	116
Twizzlers:		
Cherry, chocolate or strawberry	1 oz.	100
Licorice	1 oz.	90
U-No Bar (Cardinet's)	⅞-oz. bar	180
Whatchamacallit (Hershey's)	1.15-oz. bar	130
World Series Bar	1 oz.	128
Zagnut Bar (Clark)	.7-oz. bar	92
Zagnut Bar (Clark)	1⅜-oz. bar	213

Food and Description	Measure or Quantity	Calories
CANDY, DIETETIC:		
Carob bar, *Joan's Natural:*		
Coconut	1 section of 3-oz. bar	43
Coconut	3-oz. bar	516
Fruit & nut	1 section of 3-oz. bar	46
Fruit & nut	3-oz. bar	559
Honey bran	1 section of 3-oz. bar	40
Honey bran	3-oz. bar	487
Peanut	1 section of 3-oz. bar	43
Peanut	3-oz. bar	521
Chocolate or chocolate flavored bar:		
(Estee):		
Bittersweet	1 section of 2½-oz. bar	35
Bittersweet	2½-oz. bar	417
Coconut	1 section of 2½-oz. bar	35
Coconut	2½-oz. bar	420
Crunch	1 section of 2-oz. bar	34
Crunch	2-oz. bar	407
Fruit & nut	1 section of 2½-oz. bar	33
Fruit & nut	2½-oz. bar	398
Milk	1 section of 2½-oz. bar	34
Milk	2½-oz. bar	413
Toasted bran	1 section of 2½-oz. bar	33
Toasted bran	2½-oz. bar	398
(Featherweight)	1 piece	45
Chocolate bar with almonds (Estee) milk	1 section of 2½-oz. bar	35
Chocolate bar with almonds (Estee) milk	2½-oz. bar	415
Estee-ets, with peanuts (Estee)	1 piece	7
Gum drops (Estee) any flavor	1 piece	3
Hard candy:		
(Estee) assorted fruit or peppermint	1 piece	11
(Estee) Tropi-mix	1 piece	10
(Featherweight) assorted	1 piece	12
Mint:		
(Estee) *Esteemints*, all flavors	1 piece	4
(Sunkist):		
Mini mint	1 piece	<1

Food and Description	Measure or Quantity	Calories
Roll mint	1 piece	4
Peanut butter cup (Estee)	1 cup	50
Raisins, chocolate-covered (Estee)	1 piece	6
Rice crisp bar (Featherweight)	1 piece	50
CANNELLONI FLORENTINE, frozen (Weight Watchers) casserole	13-oz. meal	448
CANTALOUPE, cubed	½ cup	24
CAPERS (Crosse & Blackwell)	1 tsp.	2
CAP'N CRUNCH, cereal (Quaker):		
Regular	¾ cup	121
Crunchberry	¾ cup	120
Peanut butter	¾ cup	127
CARAWAY SEED (French's)	1 tsp.	8
CARNATION INSTANT BREAKFAST	1 pkg.	130
CARROT:		
Raw	5½" x 1" carrot	21
Boiled, slices	½ cup	24
Canned, regular:		
(Del Monte) drained	½ cup	35
(Libby's) solids & liq.	½ cup	20
(Stokely-Van Camp) solids & liq.	½ cup	25
Canned, dietetic:		
(Featherweight) solids & liq.	½ cup	30
(S&W) *Nutradiet,* sliced, solids & liq.	½ cup	30
(Tillie Lewis) *Tasti-Diet,* solids & liq.	½ cup	30
Frozen:		
(Birds Eye) with brown sugar glaze	⅓ pkg.	81
(Green Giant) nuggets in butter sauce	⅓ pkg.	46
(McKenzie)	⅓ pkg.	39
(Seabrook Farms)	⅓ pkg.	39
CARROT JUICE, canned (Diamond A)	½ cup	30
CARROT PUREE, canned, dietetic (Featherweight) low sodium	1 cup	70
CASABA MELON	1-lb. melon	61
CASHEW NUT:		
(Planters):		
Dry roasted	1 oz.	160

Food and Description	Measure or Quantity	Calories
Oil roasted	1 oz.	170
(Tom Houston)	15 nuts	168
CATSUP:		
Regular:		
(Del Monte)	1 T.	24
(Smucker's)	1 T.	21
Dietetic (Featherweight)	1 T.	7
CAULIFLOWER:		
Raw or boiled buds	½ cup	14
Frozen:		
(Birds Eye)	⅓ pkg.	25
(Green Giant) in cheese sauce, *Bake 'n Serve*	⅓ pkg.	80
(Mrs. Paul's) light batter & cheese	⅓ pkg.	136
(Seabrook Farms)	⅓ pkg.	23
(Stouffer's) au gratin	5-oz. serving	157
CAVIAR:		
Pressed	1 oz.	90
Whole eggs	1 T.	42
CELERY:		
1 large outer stalk	8" x 1½" at root end	7
Diced or cut	½ cup	9
Salt (French's)	1 tsp.	2
Seed (French's)	1 tsp.	11
*CELERY SOUP, cream of:		
(Ann Page)	1 cup	63
(Campbell)	10-oz. serving	120
CERTS	1 piece	6
CHABLIS WINE:		
(B&G: Inglenook-Navelle)	3 fl. oz.	60
(Gallo)	3 fl. oz.	61
(Great Western)	3 fl. oz.	70
CHAMPAGNE:		
(Bollinger)	3 fl. oz.	72
(Great Western):		
Regular	3 fl. oz.	71
Brut	3 fl. oz.	74
Extra dry	3 fl. oz.	78
Pink	3 fl. oz.	81
(Taylor) dry	3 fl. oz.	78
CHARLOTTE RUSSE, homemade recipe	4 oz.	324
*CHEDDAR CHEESE SOUP (Campbell)	11-oz. serving	180
CHEERIOS, cereal, regular or honey & nut	1 oz.	110

Food and Description	Measure or Quantity	Calories
CHEESE:		
American or cheddar:		
Natural:		
Cube	1" cube	68
Laughing Cow	1 oz.	110
Wispride, sharp	1 oz.	115
Process:		
(Borden)	¾-oz. slice	83
(Kraft)	1-oz. slice	106
Blue:		
(Frigo)	1 oz.	100
Laughing Cow	⅛-oz. cube	12
Laughing Cow	¾-oz. wedge	55
Camembert	1 oz.	85
Colby (Pauly) low sodium	1 oz.	115
Cottage (Frigo):		
Creamed, unflavored	8-oz. serving	240
Uncreamed, part skim milk	8-oz. serving	192
Cream cheese (Kraft)		
Philadelphia, plain, unwhipped	1 oz.	104
Edam:		
(House of Gold)	1 oz.	100
Laughing Cow	1 oz.	100
Farmer, *Wispride*	1 oz.	100
Gorgonzola (Foremost Blue Moon)	1 oz.	110
Gouda:		
(Foremost Blue Moon) baby	1 oz.	120
(Frigo)	1 oz.	100
Laughing Cow	1 oz.	110
Wispride	1 oz.	100
Gruyere, *Swiss Knight*	1 oz.	100
Limburger (Kraft)	1 oz.	97
Monterey Jack (Frigo)	1 oz.	100
Mozzarella (Kraft)	1 oz.	79
Muenster, natural, *Wispride*	1 oz.	100
Parmesan, grated (Kraft)	1 oz.	127
Port du Salut (Foremost Blue Moon)	1 oz.	100
Provolone:		
Laughing Cow	⅛-oz. cube	12
Laughing Cow	¾-oz. wedge	55
Laughing Cow	1-oz. serving	74
Ricotta (Frigo) part skim milk	1 oz.	43
Romano, grated (Frigo)	1 oz.	100
Roquefort (Kraft)	1 oz.	105

Food and Description	Measure or Quantity	Calories
Scamorze (Frigo)	1 oz.	79
Swiss, domestic (Kraft)	1 oz.	104
CHEESE FONDUE, *Swiss Knight*	1-oz. serving	60
CHEESE FOOD:		
American or cheddar:		
(Pauly)	.8-oz. slice	74
(Weight Watchers) colored or white	1-oz. slice	50
Wispride, cheddar:		
Regular	1 oz.	100
& blue cheese	1 oz.	100
hickory smoked	1 oz.	90
& port wine	1 oz.	90
Sharp	1 oz.	90
& swiss cheese	1 oz.	100
Cheez-ola (Fisher)	1 oz.	70
Pimiento (Pauly)	.8-oz. slice	73
Swiss (Pauly)	.8-oz. slice	74
CHEESE PUFFS, frozen (Durkee)	1 piece	59
CHEESE SPREAD:		
American or cheddar:		
(Fisher)	1 oz.	80
(Nabisco) *Snack Mate*	1 tsp.	16
(Pauly)	.8-oz. serving	71
Wispride, sharp	1 oz.	80
Cheese 'n Bacon (Nabisco) *Snack Mate*	1 tsp.	16
Cheez Whiz	1 oz.	78
Count Down (Fisher)	1 oz.	30
Imitation (Fisher) *Chef's Delight*	1 oz.	40
Pimiento:		
(Nabisco) *Snack Mate*	1 tsp.	15
(Price's)	1 oz.	80
Sharp (Pauly)	.8 oz.	77
Swiss, process (Pauly)	.8-oz.	76
Velveeta (Kraft)	1 oz.	85
CHEESE STRAW, frozen (Durkee)	1 piece	29
CHENIN BLANC WINE (Inglenook)	3 fl. oz.	60
CHERRY, sweet:		
Fresh, with stems	½ cup	41
Canned, regular (Stokely-Van Camp) pitted, solids & liq.	½ cup	50
Canned, dietetic, solids & liq.:		
(Diet Delight) with pits, water pack	½ cup	73

Food and Description	Measure or Quantity	Calories
(Featherweight) dark, water pack	½ cup	60
(Featherweight) light, water pack	½ cup	50
(Tillie Lewis) *Tasti-Diet*, light	½ cup	58
CHERRY, CANDIED	1 oz.	96
CHERRY DRINK:		
Canned:		
(Ann Page)	1 cup	124
(Hi-C)	6 fl. oz.	93
(Lincoln) cherry berry	6 fl. oz.	95
*Mix (Hi-C)	6 fl. oz.	72
CHERRY HEERING (Hiram Walker)	1 fl. oz.	80
CHERRY JELLY:		
Sweetened (Smucker's)	1 T.	53
Dietetic:		
(Featherweight)	1 T.	16
(Featherweight) artificially sweetened	1 T.	6
(Slenderella)	1 T.	24
CHERRY LIQUEUR (DeKuyper)	1 fl. oz.	75
CHERRY PRESERVE OR JAM:		
Sweetened (Smucker's)	1 T.	53
Dietetic:		
(Dia-Mel)	1 tsp.	2
(Featherweight) red	1 T.	16
(S&W) *Nutradiet*, red, tart	1 T.	12
CHERRY SPREAD, low sugar (Smucker's)	1 T.	24
CHESTNUT, fresh, in shell	¼ lb.	178
CHEWING GUM:		
Sweetened:		
Bazooka, bubble	1¢ slice	18
Beechies, Chicklets, tiny size	1 piece	6
Beech Nut; Beeman's; Big Red; Black Jack; Clove; Doublemint; Freedent; Fruit Punch; Juicy Fruit; Spearmint (Wrigley's); *Teaberry*	1 stick	10
Dentyne	1 piece	4
Dietetic:		
Bazooka, sugarless	1 piece	16
(Clark; *Care*Free*)	1 piece	7
(Estee) bubble or regular	1 piece	5

Food and Description	Measure or Quantity	Calories
(Featherweight) bubble or regular	1 piece	4
CHIANTI WINE:		
(Antinori) Classico, of 1955 or vintage	3 fl. oz.	87
(Italian Swiss Colony)	3 fl. oz.	83
(Louis M. Martini)	3 fl. oz.	90
CHICKARINA SOUP (Progresso)	1 cup	100
CHICKEN:		
Broiler, cooked, meat only	3 oz.	116
Fryer, fried, meat & skin	3 oz.	212
Fryer, fried, meat only	3 oz.	178
Fryer, fried, a 2½ lb. chicken (weighed with bone before cooking) will give you:		
Back	1 back	139
Breast	½ breast	154
Leg or drumstick	1 leg	87
Neck	1 neck	121
Rib	1 rib	42
Thigh	1 thigh	118
Wing	1 wing	78
Fried skin	1 oz.	119
Hen & cock:		
Stewed, meat & skin	3 oz.	269
Stewed, dark meat only	3 oz.	176
Stewed, light meat only	3 oz.	153
Stewed, diced	½ cup	139
Roaster, roasted, dark or light meat without skin	3 oz.	156
CHICKEN A LA KING:		
Home recipe	1 cup	468
Canned:		
(Richardson & Robbins)	1 cup	272
(Swanson)	½ of 10½-oz. can	180
Frozen:		
(Banquet)	5-oz. bag	138
(Green Giant) *Toast Topper*	5-oz. pkg.	162
(Stouffer's) with rice	½ of 9½-oz. pkg.	165
CHICKEN BOUILLON:		
(Croyden House)	1 tsp.	12
(Herb-Ox)	1 cube	6
(Herb-Ox) instant	1 packet	12
(Maggi)	1 cube	7
MBT	1 packet	12
CHICKEN, BONED, CANNED:		
(Hormel) chunk	6¾-oz. serving	257

Food and Description	Measure or Quantity	Calories
(Swanson) chunk:		
Mixin chicken	2½-oz.	120
Thigh	2½-oz.	120
White	2½-oz.	110
CHICKEN, CREAMED, frozen (Stouffer's)	6½ oz.	300
CHICKEN CROQUETTE DINNER, frozen (Morton)	10¼-oz. dinner	413
CHICKEN DINNER OR ENTREE:		
Canned (Swanson) & dumplings	7½ oz.	230
Frozen:		
(Banquet):		
& dumplings	2-lb. buffet bag	1209
& dumplings	12-oz. dinner	282
Man Pleaser	17-oz. dinner	1028
(Green Giant):		
& biscuits	7-oz. serving	196
& biscuits, *Bake'n Serve*	7-oz. entree	200
& noodles, boil-in-bag	8-oz. bag	250
(Morton):		
Boneless	10-oz. dinner	222
Boneless, king size	17-oz. dinner	546
Country Table	15-oz. dinner	682
Country Table	15-oz. dinner	682
Country Table, fried	12-oz. entree	583
& dumplings	11-oz. dinner	272
Fried	11-oz. dinner	450
(Stouffer's):		
Cacciatore, with spaghetti	11¼-oz. meal	313
Divan	8½-oz. serving	336
(Swanson):		
Hungry Man:		
Fried	15¾-oz. dinner	910
Fried	12-oz. entree	620
Fried, barbecue flavor	16½-oz. dinner	760
Fried, barbecue flavor	12-oz. entree	550
TV Brand		
Fried	11½-oz. dinner	560
Fried, barbecue flavor	11¼-oz. dinner	530
Fried, crispy	10¾-oz. dinner	650
Fried, with whipped potatoes	7-oz. entree	360
Nibbles, with french fries	6-oz. entree	370
3-course, fried	15-oz. dinner	630
In white wine sauce	8¼-oz. entree	370
(Weight Watchers):		
Creole, casserole	13-oz. meal	256

Food and Description	Measure or Quantity	Calories
Divan	9-oz. meal	210
With liver & onion	10½-oz. meal	210
Oriental style	15-oz. meal	346
With stuffing	16-oz. meal	411
White meat	9-oz. meal	291
CHICKEN FRICASSEE, canned (Richardson & Robbins)	1 cup	256
CHICKEN, FRIED, frozen		
(Banquet)	11-oz. pkg.	530
(Banquet)	2-lb. bag	2591
(Morton)	2-lb. pkg.	1490
(Morton) breast portion	21-oz. pkg.	1468
(Swanson):		
Assorted pieces	3.2-oz. serving	260
Breast	3.2-oz. serving	250
Nibbles (wing)	3.2-oz. serving	290
Take-out style	4-oz. serving	260
Thighs & drumsticks	3.2-oz. serving	260
CHICKEN LIVER PUFF, frozen (Durkee)	½-oz. piece	48
CHICKEN & NOODLES:		
Canned (College Inn)	5-oz. serving	170
Frozen:		
(Banquet) buffet	1-lb. pkg.	764
(Green Giant)	9-oz. pkg.	246
(Stouffer's):		
Escalloped	5¾-oz. serving	252
Paprikash	10½-oz. serving	391
CHICKEN PARMIGIANA, frozen (Weight Watchers)		
CHICKEN PIE, frozen:		
(Banquet)	8-oz. pie	427
(Morton)	8-oz. pie	345
(Stouffer's)	10-oz. pie	493
(Swanson)	8-oz. pie	450
(Swanson) *Hungry Man*	1-lb. pie	780
(Van de Kamp's)	7½-oz. pie	520
CHICKEN PUFF (Durkee)	½-oz. piece	49
CHICKEN SALAD (Carnation)	1½-oz. serving	94
CHICKEN SOUP:		
Canned, regular:		
*(Ann Page):		
Cream of	1 cup	104
& noodle	1 cup	66
& rice	1 cup	47

Food and Description	Measure or Quantity	Calories
(Campbell):		
Chunky:		
Regular	10¾-oz. can	230
Rice	19-oz. can	300
Vegetable	19-oz. can	380
*Condensed:		
Alphabet	10-oz. serving	110
Broth	10-oz. serving	50
Broth & noodles	10-oz. serving	80
Broth & rice	10-oz. serving	60
Broth & vegetables	10-oz. serving	30
Cream of	10-oz. serving	140
Creamy, mushroom	10-oz. serving	150
'N dumplings	10-oz. serving	100
Gumbo	10-oz. serving	70
Noodle	10-oz. serving	90
Noodle-O's	10-oz. serving	90
Rice	10-oz. serving	80
& stars	10-oz. serving	80
Vegetable	10-oz. serving	90
*Semi-condensed, *Soup for One:*		
& noodle	7¾-oz. can	130
Vegetable, full-flavored	7¾-oz. can	130
(College Inn) broth	1 cup	35
(Swanson) broth	7¼-oz. serving	35
Canned, dietetic:		
(Campbell) *Chunky*, low sodium	7½-oz. can	160
*(Dia-Mel) & noodle	8-oz. serving	50
(Featherweight) & noodle	8-oz. serving	120
(Slim-ette) broth	8-oz. serving	7
*Mix:		
(Lipton):		
Broth, *Cup-a-Broth*	6 fl. oz.	25
Cream of, *Cup-a-Soup*	1 pkg.	80
Giggle Noodle	1 cup	80
& noodle, with meat	1 cup	70
& rice	1 cup	60
(Nestlé) *Souptime:*		
Cream of	6 fl. oz.	100
& noodle	6 fl. oz.	30
CHICKEN SPREAD:		
(Swanson)	1 oz. serving	70
(Underwood)	1-oz. serving	63

Food and Description	Measure or Quantity	Calories
CHICKEN STEW, canned:		
Regular:		
(B&M)	1 cup	128
(Bounty)	7½-oz. serving	175
(Libby's) with dumplings	8-oz. serving	200
(Swanson)	½ of 15¼-oz. can	182
Dietetic:		
(Dia-Mel)	8-oz. can	150
(Featherweight)	7¼-oz. can	160
CHICORY, WITLOOF, cut	½ cup	4
CHILI or CHILI CON CARNE:		
Canned with beans:		
(Armour Star)	7¼-oz. serving	346
(Campbell) low sodium	7¾-oz. serving	310
(Hormel)	7½-oz. serving	321
(Hormel) *Short Orders*, regular or hot	7½-oz. can	300
(Libby's)	7½-oz. serving	293
(Morton House)	7½-oz. serving	340
(Nalley's)	8-oz. serving	314
(Swanson)	7¾-oz. serving	310
Canned without beans:		
(Hormel)	7½-oz. serving	345
(Hormel) *Short Orders*	7½-oz. can	370
(Libby's)	7½-oz. serving	276
(Morton House)	7½-oz. serving	340
(Nalley's)	8-oz. serving	209
(Nalley's) *Big Chunk*	7½-oz. can	383
Frozen (Stouffer's) with beans	8¾-oz. serving	272
CHILI BEEF SOUP (Campbell):		
Chunky	11-oz. can	300
*Condensed	11-oz. serving	180
CHILI SAUCE:		
(Ortega) green	1 oz.	6
(Featherweight) dietetic	1 T.	8
CHILI SEASONING MIX:		
*(Durkee)	1 cup	465
(French's) *Chili-O*	1 pkg.	150
CHOCOLATE, BAKING:		
(Hershey's):		
Bitter	1 oz.	188
Chips, dark	1 oz.	151
Chips, milk	1 oz.	148
(Nestlé):		
Choco-Bake, premelted, unsweetened	1-oz. packet	170
Morsels, milk or semisweet	1 oz.	150

Food and Description	Measure or Quantity	Calories
CHOCOLATE, HOT, home recipe	1 cup	238
CHOCOLATE ICE CREAM:		
(Meadow Gold)	¼ pint	140
(Prestige) French	¼ pint	182
(Swift's)	½ cup	129
CHOCOLATE SYRUP (See SYRUP, Chocolate)		
CHOP SUEY:		
Canned (Hung's):		
Chicken	8-oz. serving	120
Meatless	8-oz. serving	112
Frozen:		
(Banquet)	12-oz. dinner	282
(Banquet) beef	7-oz. bag	73
(Stouffer's) beef, with rice	12-oz. serving	355
Mix:		
(Durkee)	1⅝-oz. pkg.	128
*(Durkee)	1¾ cups	557
CHOWDER, canned:		
Beef & vegetable (Hormel)	7½ oz. can	120
Chicken 'n corn (Hormel)	7½-oz. can	130
Clam:		
Manhattan style:		
(Campbell) *Chunky*	19-oz. can	320
*(Campbell) condensed	10-oz. serving	90
(Crosse & Blackwell)	6½-oz. serving	50
(Progresso)	1 cup	100
New England style:		
*(Campbell):		
Condensed, made with milk	10-oz. serving	200
Condensed, made with water	10-oz. serving	100
Semicondensed, *Soup For One*, made with milk	7¾-oz. can	190
Semicondensed, *Soup For One*, made with water	7¾-oz. can	120
(Crosse & Blackwell)	6½-oz. serving	90
Ham & potato (Hormel)	7½-oz. can	130
CHOW MEIN:		
Canned:		
(Chun King):		
Chicken	8-oz. serving	60
Pork, *Divider-Pak*	12-oz. serving	110
(Hormel) pork, *Short Orders*	7½-oz. can	140
(La Choy):		
Beef	1 cup	72

Food and Description	Measure or Quantity	Calories
*Beef, bi-pack	1 cup	83
Chicken	½ of 1-lb. can	68
*Chicken, bi-pack	1 cup	101
Meatless	1 cup	47
*Mushroom, bi-pack	1 cup	85
Pepper Oriental	1 cup	89
*Pepper Oriental, bi-pack	1 cup	89
*Pork, bi-pack	1 cup	120
Shrimp	1 cup	61
*Shrimp, bi-pack	1 cup	110
Frozen:		
(Banquet) chicken	7-oz. bag	89
(Chun King):		
Chicken	11-oz. dinner	320
Shrimp	11-oz. dinner	300
(Green Giant) chicken	9-oz. entree	126
(La Choy):		
Beef, 5-compartment	11-oz. dinner	337
Beef, entree	8-oz. serving	97
Chicken	11-oz. dinner	356
Chicken	8-oz. entree	108
Pepper Oriental	11-oz. dinner	332
Pepper Oriental	7½-oz. entree	103
Shrimp	11-oz. dinner	323
Shrimp	8-oz. entree	73
(Stouffer's) chicken	8-oz. serving	145
CHUTNEY (Major Grey's)	1 T.	53
CINNAMON, GROUND (French's)	1 tsp.	6
CITRUS COOLER DRINK, canned:		
(Ann Page)	1 cup	118
(Hi-C)	6 fl. oz.	93
CLAM:		
Raw, all kinds, meat only	1 cup (8 oz.)	59
Raw, soft, meat & liq.	1 lb. (weighed in shell)	142
Canned (Doxsee):		
Chopped & minced, solids & liq.	4 oz.	59
Chopped, meat only	4 oz.	111
Frozen (Mrs. Paul's):		
Deviled	3-oz. piece	179
Fried	2½ oz.	264
CLAMATO COCKTAIL (Mott's)	6 fl. oz.	80
CLAM CAKE, thins (Mrs. Paul's)	2½-oz. piece	158
CLAM CHOWDER (See CHOWDER, Clam)		

Food and Description	Measure or Quantity	Calories
CLAM JUICE (Snow)	½ cup	15
CLAM STICK, breaded (Mrs. Paul's)	.8-oz. piece	49
CLARET WINE:		
(Gold Seal)	3 fl. oz.	82
(Inglenook) Navelle	3 fl. oz.	60
(Taylor) 12.5% alcohol	3 fl. oz.	72
CLORETS, gum or mint	1 piece	6
COCOA:		
Dry, unsweetened:		
(Droste)	1 T.	21
(Hershey's)	1 T.	29
(Sultana)	1 T.	30
Mix, regular:		
(Alba '66) instant, all flavors	1 envelope	60
(Carnation) all flavors	1-oz. pkg.	112
(Hershey's):		
Hot	1 oz.	110
Instant	3 T.	76
(Nestlé):		
Hot	1 oz.	110
With mini marshmallows	1 oz.	110
(Ovaltine) hot	1.1-oz. pkg.	130
Swiss Miss	1 oz.	112
Swiss Miss, instant, with mini marshmallows	1.1-oz.	123
Mix, dietetic:		
(Ovaltine) hot, reduced calorie	.45-oz. pkg.	50
Swiss Miss, instant, lite	3 T.	70
COCOA KRISPIES, cereal	¾ cup	110
COCOA PUFFS, cereal	1 oz.	110
COCONUT:		
Fresh, meat only	2" x 2" x ½" piece	156
Grated or shredded, loosely packed	½ cup	225
Dried:		
(Baker's):		
Angel Flake	¼ cup	95
Cookie	¼ cup	137
Premium shredded	¼ cup	100
(Durkee) shredded	¼ cup	69
COCO WHEATS, cereal	1 T.	44
COD, broiled	3 oz.	144

Food and Description	Measure or Quantity	Calories
COFFEE:		
Regular:		
Max-Pax; Maxwell House Electra Perk; Yuban; Yuban Electra Matic	6 fl. oz.	2
Mellow Roast	6 fl. oz.	8
Decaffeinated:		
Brim, regular or electric perk	6 fl. oz.	2
Brim, freeze-dried	6 fl. oz.	4
Decaf	6 fl. oz.	4
Nescafé, freeze-dried	6 fl. oz.	4
Sanka, regular or electric perk	6 fl. oz.	2
Freeze-dried, Maxim, Sanka, Taster's Choice	6 fl. oz.	4
Instant:		
*(Chase & Sanborn)	5 fl. oz.	1
Decaf (Nestlé)	6 fl. oz.	4
Mellow Roast	6 fl. oz.	8
Nescafé	6 fl. oz.	4
Sunrise	6 fl. oz.	6
Mix (General Foods): Cafe Francais, Cafe Vienna, Irish Mocha Mint, Orange Cappuccino, Suisse Mocha	6 fl. oz.	60
COFFEE CAKE (See CAKE, Coffee)		
COFFEE LIQUEUR (DeKuyper)	1½ fl. oz.	140
COFFEE SOUTHERN	1 fl. oz.	79
COLA SOFT DRINK (See SOFT DRINK, Cola)		
COLD DUCK WINE (Great Western) pink	3 fl. oz.	92
COLESLAW, solids & liq., made with mayonnaise-type salad dressing	1 cup	118
COLLARDS:		
Leaves, cooked	½ cup	31
Frozen:		
(Birds Eye) chopped	⅓ pkg.	25
(Stouffer's) chopped	⅓ pkg.	31
CONCORD WINE:		
(Gold Seal)	3 fl. oz.	125
(Mogen David)	3 fl. oz.	120
(Pleasant Valley) red	3 fl. oz.	90

Food and Description	Measure or Quantity	Calories
CONSOMMÉ MADRILENE (Crosse & Blackwell):		
Clear	6½ oz.	25
Red	6½ oz.	30
COOKIE, REGULAR:		
Almond windmill (Nabisco)	1 piece	47
Animal cracker:		
(Nabisco) *Barnum's Animals*	1 piece	12
(Sunshine) iced	1 piece	26
Apple Crisp (Nabisco)	1 piece	50
Assortment (Nabisco) *Mayfair*:		
Crown creme sandwich	1 piece	53
Fancy shortbread biscuit	1 piece	22
Filigree creme sandwich	1 piece	60
Mayfair creme sandwich	1 piece	65
Tea rose creme	1 piece	53
Tea time biscuit	1 piece	25
Biscos (Nabisco)	1 piece	43
Bordeaux (Pepperidge Farm)	1 piece	36
Brown edge wafers (Nabisco)	1 piece	28
Brownie:		
(Frito-Lays) nut fudge	1.8-oz. piece	200
(Hostess)	1¼-oz. piece	159
(Sara Lee) frozen	⅛ of 13-oz. pkg.	199
Butter (Nabisco)	1 piece	23
Butterscotch chip (Nabisco) *Bakers Bonus*	1 piece	80
Caramel peanut log (Nabisco) *Heydey*	1 piece	120
Cheda-Nut (Nabisco)	1 piece	38
Cheese peanut-butter (Nabisco)	1 piece	35
Chocolate & chocolate-covered:		
Pinwheels (Nabisco)	1 piece	140
Wafers (Nabisco) *Famous*	1 piece	28
Chocolate chip:		
Chips Ahoy! (Nabisco)	1 piece	53
Cookie Little (Nabisco)	1 piece	7
Cinnamon Treats (Nabisco)	1 piece	27
Coconut:		
(Nabisco) bar, *Bakers Bonus*	1 piece	43
Nabisco (chocolate chip)	1 piece	75
Creme wafer stick (Nabisco)	1 piece	50
Devil's food cake (Nabisco)	1 piece	50
Double chips fudge (Nabisco)	1 piece	80
Fig bar:		
Fig Newtons (Nabisco)	1 piece	60
Fig Wheats (Nabisco)	1 piece	60

Food and Description	Measure or Quantity	Calories
Gingersnaps (Nabisco) old fashioned	1 piece	30
Ladyfinger	3¼" x 1⅜" x 1⅛"	40
Lemon (Planters) creme	1 oz.	140
Macaroon, coconut (Nabisco)	1 piece	95
Marshmallow:		
(Nabisco):		
Mallomars	1 piece	60
Puffs, cocoa covered	1 piece	85
Sandwich	1 piece	30
Twirls cakes	1 piece	130
(Planters) banana pie	1 oz.	127
Mint sandwich (Nabisco) *Mystic*	1 piece	88
Molasses (Nabisco) *Pantry*	1 piece	60
Oatmeal:		
(Nabisco)	1 piece	75
(Nabisco) *Bakers Bonus*	1 piece	80
(Nabisco) *Cookie Little*	1 piece	6
(Tastykake) raisin bar	1 pkg.	267
Party Grahams (Nabisco)	1 piece	47
Peanut & peanut butter (Nabisco):		
Creme patties	1 piece	35
Peanut brittle	1 piece	50
Piccolo	1 piece	22
Sandwich, *Nutter Butter*	1 piece	70
Raisin	1 oz.	107
Raisin (Nabisco) fruit biscuit	1 piece	60
Sandwich (Nabisco):		
Brown edge	1 piece	80
Cameo creme	1 piece	70
Cheese flavored	1 piece	27
Cookie Break, mixed	1 piece	53
Cookie Break, vanilla	1 piece	50
Gaity, fudge	1 piece	53
Mystic, mint	1 piece	90
Oreo, chocolate	1 piece	50
Oreo, Double Stuf	1 piece	70
Swiss	1 piece	50
Shortbread or shortcake (Nabisco):		
Cookie Little	1 piece	6
Lorna Doone	1 piece	40
Melt-A-Way	1 piece	70
Pecan	1 piece	80
Striped	1 piece	22

Food and Description	Measure or Quantity	Calories
Social Tea, biscuit (Nabisco)	1 piece	22
Spiced wafers (Nabisco)	1 piece	33
Sugar cookie (Nabisco) rings	1 piece	70
Sugar wafer:		
(Dutch Treat)	1 piece	49
(Dutch Twin)	1 piece	48
(Nabisco) *Biscos*	1 piece	19
Vanilla creme (Wise)	1 piece	33
Vanilla creme (Planters)	1 oz.	116
Vanilla wafer (Nabisco) *Nilla*	1 piece	19
Waffle creme (Dutch Twin)	1 piece	45
COOKIE, DIETETIC:		
Chocolate chip:		
(Estee)	1 piece	28
(Featherweight)	1 piece	40
Chocolate crescent (Featherweight)	1 piece	40
Coconut (Estee)	1 piece	25
Fudge (Estee)	1 piece	27
Lemon (Featherweight)	1 piece	40
Lemon thin (Estee)	1 piece	24
Oatmeal raisin (Estee)	1 piece	23
Sandwich:		
(Estee) duplex	1 piece	47
(Featherweight) creme	1 piece	50
Vanilla (Featherweight)	1 piece	40
Wafer:		
Chocolate-covered (Estee)	1 piece	128
Chocolate creme (Featherweight)	1 piece	40
Filled, creme, assorted (Estee)	1 piece	35
Filled, creme, chocolate or vanilla (Estee)	1 piece	24
Peanut butter creme (Featherweight)	1 piece	40
Wheat germ (Estee)	1 piece	6
Vanilla creme (Featherweight)	1 piece	40
COOKIE CRISP, cereal, any flavor	1 cup	110
***COOKIE DOUGH** (Pillsbury):*		
Chocolate chip	1 cookie	53
Oatmeal	1 cookie	57
Peanut butter	1 cookie	57
Sugar	1 cookie	60

Food and Description	Measure or Quantity	Calories
*COOKIE MIX:		
Regular:		
Brownie:		
(Betty Crocker) fudge, regular size	1/16 of pan	150
(Betty Crocker) German chocolate	1/16 of pan	150
(Nestlé)	1/23 of pkg.	150
(Pillsbury) fudge, regular size	1½" square	65
Chocolate, double:		
(Betty Crocker) *Big Batch*	1 cookie	60
(Duncan Hines)	1/36 pkg.	67
Chocolate chip:		
(Betty Crocker) *Big Batch*	1 cookie	60
(Duncan Hines)	1/36 of pkg.	72
(Nestlé)	1 cookie	60
(Quaker)	1 cookie	75
Date bar (Betty Crocker)	1/32 of pkg.	60
Fudge chip (Quaker)	1 cookie	75
Macaroon, coconut (Betty Crocker)	1/24 of pkg.	80
Oatmeal:		
(Betty Crocker) *Big Batch*	1 cookie	65
(Duncan Hines) raisin	1/36 of pkg.	68
(Nestlé) raisin	1 cookie	60
(Quaker)	1 cookie	66
Peanut butter:		
(Betty Crocker) *Big Batch*	1 cookie	65
(Betty Crocker) *Big Batch*, with flavored chips	1 cookie	60
(Nestlé)	1 cookie	65
Sugar:		
(Betty Crocker) *Big Batch*	1 cookie	60
(Duncan Hines) golden	1/36 pkg.	59
(Nestlé)	1 cookie	65
Vienna dream bar (Betty Crocker)	1/24 of pkg.	90
Dietetic (Dia-Mel)	2" cookie	50
COOKING SPRAY, *Mazola No Stick*	2-second spray	7
CORN:		
Fresh, on the cob, boiled	5" x 1¾" ear	70
Canned, regular pack:		
(Del Monte):		
Cream style, golden, wet pack	½ cup	89

Food and Description	Measure or Quantity	Calories
Whole kernel, drained	½ cup	100
Whole kernel, vacuum pack	½ cup	101
(Green Giant):		
Cream style	4¼ oz.	103
Whole kernel, solids & liq.	4¼ oz.	77
Whole kernel, *Mexicorn*, solids & liq.	4 oz.	97
Whole kernel, *Niblets*, vacuum pack	4 oz.	94
(Le Sueur) solids & liq.	4¼ oz.	84
(Libby's):		
Cream style	½ cup	100
Whole kernel, solids & liq.	½ cup	92
(Stokely-Van Camp):		
Cream style	½ cup	105
Whole kernel, solids & liq.	½ cup	74
Canned, dietetic pack:		
(Diet Delight) solids & liq.	½ cup	71
(Featherweight) whole kernel, solids & liq.	½ cup	80
(S&W) *Nutradiet*, solids & liq.	½ cup	80
(Tillie Lewis) *Tasti-Diet*, solids & liq.	½ cup	70
Frozen:		
(Birds Eye):		
On the cob	4.9-oz. ear	130
On the cob, *Little Ears*	1 ear	70
Whole kernel	⅓ of pkg.	70
(Green Giant):		
On the cob	5½" ear	155
On the cob, *Nibbler*	3" ear	85
Whole kernel, golden	4 oz.	100
Whole kernel, *Mexicorn*, golden, in butter sauce	⅓ of pkg.	86
Whole kernel, white, in butter sauce	⅓ of pkg.	89
(McKenzie) on the cob	5" ear	140
(Ore-Ida):		
On the cob	1 ear	140
Whole kernel	3.2-oz. serving	106
(Seabrook Farms):		
On the cob	5" ear	140
Whole kernel	⅓ of pkg.	97
CORNBREAD:		
Home recipe:		
Corn pone	4 oz.	231
Spoon bread	4 oz.	221

Food and Description	Measure or Quantity	Calories
*Mix:		
(Aunt Jemima)	⅛ of pkg.	220
(Dromedary)	2" x 2" piece	130
(Pillsbury) *Ballard*	⅟₁₆ of recipe	160
CORN CHEX, cereal	1 cup	110
CORN DOGS, frozen:		
(Hormel)	1 weiner	230
(Hormel) *Tater Dogs*	1 weiner	190
*(Oscar Mayer)	4-oz. piece	328
CORNED BEEF:		
Cooked, boneless, medium fat	4 oz.	422
Canned:		
Dinty Moore	3-oz. serving	196
(Libby's)	3½-oz. serving	244
Packaged:		
(Eckrich) sliced	1-oz. slice	41
(Oscar Mayer) jellied loaf	1-oz. slice	44
(Vienna):		
Brisket	1-oz. serving	88
Flats	1-oz. serving	49
CORNED BEEF HASH, canned:		
(Libby's)	1 cup	454
Mary Kitchen	7½-oz. serving	399
Mary Kitchen, Short Orders	7½-oz. can	370
CORNED BEEF HASH DINNER, frozen (Banquet)	10-oz. dinner	372
CORNED BEEF SPREAD (Underwood)	1 oz.	55
CORN FLAKE CRUMBS (Kellogg's)	¼ cup	110
CORN FLAKES, cereal:		
(Featherweight) low sodium	1 cup	88
(General Mills) Country	1 cup	110
(Kellogg's)	1 cup	110
(Kellogg's) honey & nut	¾ cup	120
King Kullen, regular	1 cup	107
King Kullen, sugar toasted	⅜ cup	108
(Post) *Post Toasties*	1¼ cups	107
(Ralston Purina)	1 cup	110
(Van Brode)	1 oz.	107
(Van Brode) low sodium	1 oz.	110
(Van Brode) sugar toasted	1 oz.	108
CORN MEAL:		
Bolted (Aunt Jemima/Quaker)	3 T.	102
Degermed	¼ cup	125

Food and Description	Measure or Quantity	Calories
Mix:		
Bolted (Aunt Jemima)	1 cup	392
Degermed (Aunt Jemima)	1 cup	392
CORN SOUFFLÉ, frozen (Stouffer's)	4-oz. serving	154
CORNSTARCH (Argo; Kingsford's; Duryea)	1 tsp.	11
CORN SYRUP (See SYRUP)		
CORN TOTAL, cereal	1 cup	110
COUGH DROP:		
(Beech-Nut)	1 drop	10
(Luden's)	1 drop	9
(Pine Bros.)	1 drop	8
(Smith Brothers)	1 drop	7
COUNT CHOCULA, cereal (General Mills)	1 oz.	110
COUNTRY CRISP, cereal	¾ cup	114
CRAB:		
Fresh, steamed:		
Whole	½ lb.	101
Meat only	4 oz.	105
Canned, king crab (Icy Point; Pillar Rock)	3¾ oz.	108
Frozen (Wakefield's Alaska King)	4 oz.	96
CRAB APPLE	¼ lb.	71
CRAB APPLE JELLY (Smucker's)	1 T.	53
CRAB CAKE THINS, breaded & fried (Mrs. Paul's)	½ of 10-oz. pkg.	324
CRAB COCKTAIL (Sau-Sea)	4 oz.	80
CRAB, DEVILED, breaded & fried (Mrs. Paul's)	½ of 6-oz. pkg.	166
CRAB IMPERIAL, home recipe	1 cup	323
CRAB SOUP (Crosse & Blackwell)	6½-oz. serving	50
CRACKERS, PUFFS & CHIPS:		
American Harvest (Nabisco)	1 piece	16
Arrowroot biscuit (Nabisco)	1 piece	20
Bacon'n Dip (Nabisco)	1 piece	21
Bacon-flavored thins (Nabisco)	1 piece	11
Bacon Nips	1 oz.	147
Bakon-Snacks	1 oz.	150
Betcha Bacon	1 oz.	170
Bugles (General Mills)	1 oz.	150
Butter thins (Nabisco)	1 piece	14
Cheese flavored:		
Bops (Nalley's)	1 oz.	147
Cheddar Bitz (Frito-Lay)	1 oz.	129

Food and Description	Measure or Quantity	Calories
Cheddar triangles (Nabisco)	1 piece	9
Cheese balls (Planters)	1 oz.	160
Cheese curls (Planters)	1 oz.	138
Cheese'n Crunch (Nabisco)	1 oz.	160
Cheese filled (Frito-Lay's)	1½ oz.	203
Cheese Pixies (Wise) baked	1 oz.	155
Cheese Pixies (Wise) fried	1 oz.	158
Chee-Tos, crunchy	1 oz.	160
Chee-Tos, puffed	1 oz.	160
Cheez Balls (Planters)	1 oz.	160
Cheez Curls (Planters)	1 oz.	160
Country cheddar'n sesame (Nabisco)	1 piece	9
Parmesan Swirl (Nabisco)	1 piece	11
Sandwich (Planters)	1 piece	29
Swiss cheese (Nabisco)	1 piece	10
Tid-Bit (Nabisco)	1 oz.	150
Twists (Bachman)	1 oz.	150
Twists (Nalley's)	1 oz.	126
Chicken in a Biskit (Nabisco)	1 piece	11
Chip O'Cheddar, Flavor Kist, (Schulze and Burch)		
Chipos (General Mills)	1 oz.	150
Chippers (Nabisco)	1 piece	15
Chipsters (Nabisco)	1 piece	2
Corn chips:		
(Bachman)	1 oz.	160
Fritos	1 oz.	160
Fritos, barbecue flavor	1 oz.	150
Korkers (Nabisco)	1 piece	8
(Old London)	1 oz.	155
(Planters)	1 oz.	170
Corn Nuggets (Frito-Lay's)	1 oz.	128
Corn Nuts (Nalley's)	1 oz.	120
Corn & Sesame Chips (Nabisco)	1 piece	10
Creme Wafer Stock (Nabisco)	1 piece	47
Crown Pilot (Nabisco)	1 piece	75
Diggers (Nabisco)	1 piece	4
Dixies (Nabisco)	1 piece	8
Doo Dads (Nabisco)	1 piece	2
Escort (Nabisco)	1 piece	21
Flings (Nabisco)	1 piece	10
French onion cracker (Nabisco)	1 piece	12
Goldfish (Pepperidge Farm):		
Thins	1 piece	17
Tiny	¼ oz.	35

Food and Description	Measure or Quantity	Calories
Graham:		
Cinnamon Treat (Nabisco)	1 piece	28
Flavor Kist (Schulze and Burch) sugar-honey coated	1 piece	57
Honey Maid (Nabisco)	1 piece	30
(Nabisco)	1 piece	30
Graham, chocolate or cocoa-covered:		
Fancy Dip (Nabisco)	1 piece	65
(Nabisco)	1 piece	57
Lil' Loaf (Nabisco)	1 piece	14
Melba Toast (See MELBA TOAST)		
Mucho Macho Nacho, Flavor Kist, (Schulze and Burch)	1 oz.	121
Munchos	1 oz.	154
Oyster, Dandy or Oysterettes (Nabisco)	1 piece	3
Ritz (Nabisco)	1 piece	17
Royal Lunch (Nabisco)	1 piece	55
Rusk, Holland (Nabisco)	1 piece	40
Ry-Krisp, natural	1 triple cracker	25
Ry-Krisp, seasoned	1 triple cracker	30
Rye wafers (Nabisco)	1 piece	23
Saltine:		
Flavor Kist (Schulze and Burch)	1 piece	12
Hi-Ho (Sunshine)	1 piece	18
Premium (Nabisco)	1 piece	12
Sea rounds (Nabisco)	1 piece	45
Sesame:		
Butter flavored (Nabisco)	1 piece	17
Sesame Wheatsl (Nabisco)	1 piece	17
Sesame wheat snack, Flavor Kist (Schulze and Burch)	1 oz.	134
Teeko (Nabisco)	1 piece	22
Skittle Chips (Nabisco)	1 piece	14
Snackin' Crisp (Durkee) O & C	1 oz.	155
Snacks Ahoy (Nabisco)	1 piece	9
Snacks sticks (Pepperidge Farm):		
Lightly salted	1 oz.	120
Pumpernickel	1 oz.	110
Sesame	1 oz.	120
Wheat	1 oz.	110
Taco chips (Nalley's)	1 oz.	147

Food and Description	Measure or Quantity	Calories
Taco corn chip (Old London)	1 oz.	133
Tater Puffs (Nabisco)	1 piece	7
Tortillo chips:		
(Bachman) nacho or taco flavor	1 oz.	150
Buenos (Nabisco) nacho flavor	1 piece	10
Buenos (Nabisco) taco flavor	1 piece	11
Doritos, nacho or taco flavor	1 oz.	140
(Nabisco) regular and nacho flavor	1 piece	11
(Nalley's)	1 oz.	147
(Planter's) nacho or taco flavor	1 oz.	130
Tostitos	1 oz.	140
Triscuit (Nabisco)	1 piece	20
Twigs (Nabisco)	1 piece	14
Uneeda Biscuit (Nabisco)	1 piece	22
Vegetable thins (Nabisco)	1 piece	11
Waverly Wafer (Nabisco)	1 piece	18
Wheat Chips (Nabisco)	1 piece	4
Wheat snack, *Flavor Kist* (Schulze and Burch):		
Regular	1 oz.	138
Rye	1 oz.	130
Wild onion	1 oz.	125
Wheatsworth (Nabisco)	1 piece	14
Wheat Thins (Nabisco)	1 piece	9
CRACKER CRUMBS, graham (Nabisco)	⅛ of 9" pie shell	70
CRACKER MEAL (Nabisco)	½ cup	220
*****CRANAPPLE JUICE** (Ocean Spray) frozen	6 fl. oz.	119
CRANBERRY, fresh (Ocean Spray)	½ cup	26
*****CRANBERRY JUICE COCKTAIL**, frozen (Ocean Spray)	6 fl. oz.	112
CRANBERRY-ORANGE JUICE DRINK (Ocean Spray)	6 fl. oz.	101
CRANBERRY-ORANGE RELISH (Ocean Spray)	1 T.	33
CRANBERRY-RASPBERRY SAUCE (Ocean Spray) jellied	2-oz. serving	85
CRANBERRY SAUCE:		
Home recipe	4 oz.	202
Canned (Ocean Spray):		
Jellied	2-oz. serving	89
Whole berry	2-oz. serving	89

Food and Description	Measure or Quantity	Calories
CRANGRAPE (Ocean Spray)	6 fl. oz.	108
*CRANORANGE JUICE DRINK, frozen (Ocean Spray)	6 fl. oz.	107
CRAZY COW, cereal (General Mills)	1 cup	110
CREAM:		
Half & Half:		
(Dean)	1 T.	22
(Meadow Gold) 12.8% fat	1 T.	30
Light, table or coffee (Sealtest) 16% fat	1 T.	26
Light, whipping, 30% fat (Sealtest)	1 T.	45
Heavy whipping (Meadow Gold)	1 T.	51
Sour:		
(Dean)	1 T.	28
Sour, imitation:		
(Pet)	1 T.	25
Sour Slim (Dean)	1 T.	30
Substitute (See CREAM SUBSTITUTE)		
CREAMIES (Tastykake):		
Chocolate	1 piece	257
Spice	1 piece	272
CREAM PUFFS, custard filling, home recipe	3½" x 2" piece	303
CREAMSICLE (Popsicle Industries)	2½-fl.-oz. piece	80
CREAM SUBSTITUTE:		
Coffee-mate; Cremora; Pream	1 tsp.	11
Coffee Rich	½ oz.	22
Coffee Twin	½ fl. oz.	18
Dairy Light (Alba)	2.8-oz. envelope	10
Half & Half (Meadow Gold)	1 T.	27
N-Rich	1½ tsp.	15
Perx	1 tsp.	8
(Pet)	1 tsp.	10
Poly Perx	½ oz.	20
(Sanna)	1 plastic cup	24
CREAM OF WHEAT, cereal:		
*Instant	¾ cup	100
Mix'n Eat, dry:		
Regular	1 packet	100
Baked apple & cinnamon	1 packet	130
Banana & spice	1 packet	130
Maple & brown sugar	3¾ T.	130

Food and Description	Measure or Quantity	Calories
Quick	2½ T.	100
Regular	2½ T.	100
CREME DE BANANA LIQUEUR		
(Mr. Boston)	1 fl. oz.	93
CREME DE CAÇAO:		
(Garnier)	1 fl. oz.	97
(Hiram Walker)	1 fl. oz.	104
(Mr. Boston):		
Brown	1 fl. oz.	103
White	1 fl. oz.	93
CREME DE CASSIS:		
(Garnier)	1 fl. oz.	83
(Mr. Boston)	1 fl. oz.	85
CREME DE MENTHE:		
(Bols)	1 fl. oz.	122
(Hiram Walker)	1 fl. oz.	94
(Mr. Boston)		
Green	1 fl. oz.	109
White	1 fl. oz.	97
CREME DE NOYAUX (Mr. Boston)	1 fl. oz.	99
CREPE, frozen:		
(Mrs. Paul's):		
Clam	5½-oz. pkg.	286
Crab	5½-oz. pkg.	247
Scallop	5½-oz. pkg.	220
Shrimp	5½-oz. pkg.	252
(Stouffer's):		
Beef burgundy	6¼-oz. pkg.	335
Chicken with mushroom sauce	8¼-oz. pkg.	390
Ham & asparagus	6¼-oz. pkg.	325
Mushroom	6¼-oz. pkg.	255
CRISP RICE, cereal:		
Breakfast Best	1 cup	107
Breakfast Best, sugar toasted	⅝ cup	108
(Ralston Purina)	1 cup	110
(Van Brode)	1 cup	107
(Van Brode) cocoa	¾ cup	108
CRISPY WHEATS'N RAISINS, cereal (General Mills)	¾ cup	110
CROQUETTES, frozen, seafood (Mrs. Paul's)	3-oz. serving	181
CROUTON:		
(Arnold):		
American or Danish style	½ oz.	66
Bavarian or English style	½ oz.	65

Food and Description	Measure or Quantity	Calories
French, Italian or Mexican style	½ oz.	66
Croutettes (Kellogg's)	⅔ cup	70
CUCUMBER:		
Eaten with skin	½-lb. cucumber	32
Pared, 10-oz. cucumber	7½" x 2" pared	29
Pared	3 slices	4
CUMIN SEED (French's)	1 tsp.	7
CUPCAKE:		
Regular:		
(Hostess):		
Chocolate	1 cupcake	166
Orange	1 cupcake	149
Tastykake:		
Chocolate	1 cupcake	100
Chocolate, creme filled	1 cupcake	122
Frozen (Sara Lee) yellow	1 cupcake	190
*CUPCAKE MIX (Flako)	1 cupcake	150
CUP O'NOODLES (Nissin Foods):		
Beef	2½-oz. serving	343
Beef, twin pack	1.2-oz. serving	151
Beef onion	2½-oz. serving	323
Beef onion, twin pack	1.2-oz. serving	158
Chicken	2½-oz. serving	343
Chicken, twin pack	1.2-oz. serving	155
Pork	2½-oz. serving	331
Shrimp	2½-oz. serving	336
CURAÇAO:		
(Bols)	1 fl. oz.	105
(Hiram Walker)	1 fl. oz.	96
CURRANT, dried, Zante (Del Monte)	½ cup	204
CURRANT JELLY (Smucker's)	1 T.	53
CUSTARD:		
Chilled, *Swiss Miss*, custard or egg flavor	4-oz. container	160
*Mix, dietetic (Featherweight)	½ cup	80
C.W. POST, cereal:		
Family-style	¼ cup	131
Family-style, with raisins	¼ cup	128

Food and Description	Measure or Quantity	Calories

D

DAIQUIRI COCKTAIL, canned (Mr. Boston):		
Regular	3 fl. oz.	99
Strawberry	3 fl. oz.	111
DATE:		
Whole (Cal-Date)	.8-oz. date	62
Imported Iraq:		
(Bordo)	.2-oz. average date	18
(Bordo) dried	¼ cup	159
DE CHAUNAC WINE (Great Western) 12% alcohol	3 fl. oz.	71
DELAWARE WINE (Gold Seal) 12% alcohol	3 fl. oz.	87
DILL SEED (French's)	1 tsp.	9
DING DONG (Hostess)	1 cake	170
DINNER, frozen (See individual listings such as BEEF, CHICKEN, TURKEY, etc.)		
DIP:		
Avocado (Nalley's)	1 oz.	114
Bacon & onion (Nalley's)	1 oz.	114
Barbecue (Nalley's)	1 oz.	114
Blue Cheese:		
(Dean) tang	1 oz.	61
(Nalley's)	1 oz.	110
Cheese-bacon (Nalley's)	1 oz.	119
Clam (Nalley's)	1 oz.	101
Cucumber & onion (Breakstone)	1 oz.	50
Dill pickle (Nalley's)	1 oz.	86
Enchilada, Fritos	1 oz.	37
Garlic (Nalley's)	1 oz.	120
Guacamole (Nalley's)	1 oz.	114
Jalapeno:		
Fritos	1 oz.	34
(Hain) natural	1 oz.	40
Onion (Dean) French	1 oz.	58
Onion bean (Hain) natural	1 oz.	41
Ranch House (Nalley's)	1 oz.	121
DISTILLED LIQUOR, any brand:		
80 proof	1 fl. oz.	65
86 proof	1 fl. oz.	70
90 proof	1 fl. oz.	74

Food and Description	Measure or Quantity	Calories
94 proof	1 fl. oz.	77
100 proof	1 fl. oz.	83
DOUGHNUT:		
Regular (Hostess):		
Cinnamon	1-oz. piece	111
Crunch	1-oz. piece	105
Enrobed	1-oz. piece	136
Old fashioned	1½-oz. piece	177
Powdered	1-oz. piece	117
Frozen (Morton):		
Bavarian creme	2-oz. piece	180
Boston creme	2.3-oz. piece	208
Chocolate iced	1½-oz. piece	148
Glazed	1½-oz. piece	150
Jelly	1.8-oz. piece	175
Mini	1.1-oz. piece	122
DRAMBUIE (Hiram Walker)	1 fl. oz.	110
DUMPLINGS, canned, dietetic (Dia-Mel) stuffed with chicken	8-oz. serving	200

E

Food and Description	Measure or Quantity	Calories
ECLAIR:		
Home recipe, with custard filling and chocolate icing	4-oz. piece	271
Frozen (Rich's) chocolate	1 piece	234
EEL, smoked, meat only	4 oz.	374
EGG, CHICKEN		
Raw, white only	1 large egg	17
Raw, yolk only	1 large egg	59
Boiled	1 large egg	81
Fried in butter	1 large egg	99
Omelet, mixed with milk & cooked in fat	1 large egg	107
Poached	1 large egg	78
Scrambled, mixed with milk & cooked in fat	1 large egg	111
*****EGG FOO YOUNG** (Chun King) stir fry	⅛ of pkg.	45
EGG MIX (Durkee):		
Omelet:		
*With bacon	½ of pkg.	310
*Puffy	½ of pkg.	302
Scrambled:		
Plain	.8-oz. pkg.	124
With bacon	1.3-oz. pkg.	181

Food and Description	Measure or Quantity	Calories
EGG NOG, dairy (Meadow Gold) 6% fat	½ cup	164
EGG NOG COCKTAIL (Mr. Boston) 15% alcohol	3 fl. oz.	180
EGGPLANT:		
Boiled	4 oz.	189
Frozen:		
(Mrs. Paul's)		
Parmesan	5½-oz. serving	259
Slices, breaded & fried	4½-oz. serving	199
Sticks, breaded & fried	3½-oz. serving	262
(Weight Watchers) parmigiana	12-oz. meal	251
EGG ROLL, frozen:		
(Chun King):		
Chicken	½-oz. roll	23
Meat & Shrimp	½-oz. roll	25
Shrimp	½-oz. roll	23
(La Choy):		
Chicken	.4-oz. roll	30
Lobster	.4-oz. roll	27
Meat & shrimp	.2-oz. roll	17
Meat & shrimp	.4-oz. roll	27
Shrimp	.4-oz. roll	26
Shrimp	2½-oz. roll	108
EGG, SCRAMBLED, frozen (Swanson) and sausage with hashed brown potatoes, TV Brand	6½-oz. entree	460
EGG SUBSTITUTE:		
Egg Beaters (Fleischmann)	¼ cup	40
Eggstra (Tillie Lewis) Tasti-Diet	1 egg	54
Scramblers (Morningstar Farms)	1 egg	33
Second Nature (Avoset)	3 T.	38
ELDERBERRY JELLY (Smucker's)	1 T.	53
ENCHILADA, frozen:		
Beef (Banquet):		
With sauce	6-oz. bag	207
With cheese & chili gravy	2-lb. pkg.	1118
Cheese:		
(Patio)	4-oz. serving	130
(Van de Kamp's) with sauce	7½-oz. serving	330
Chicken (Van de Kamp's) with sauce	7½-oz. serving	270
ENCHILADA DINNER, frozen:		
Beef:		
(Banquet)	12-oz. dinner	479

Food and Description	Measure or Quantity	Calories
(Morton)	12-oz. dinner	351
(Swanson) TV Brand	15-oz. dinner	570
(Van de Kamp's)	12-oz. dinner	420
Cheese:		
(Banquet)	12-oz. dinner	459
(Van de Kamp's)	12-oz. dinner	430
*ENCHILADA SAUCE MIX		
(Durkee)	1 cup	57
ENDIVE, CURLY, or ESCAROLE, cut up	½ cup	7
ESCARCLE SOUP, canned (Progresso) in chicken broth	6-oz. serving	25
EXPRESSO COFFEE LIQUEUR	1 fl. oz.	104

F

FARINA:		
(Hi-O) dry, regular	¼ cup	157
Malt-O-Meal, dry, regular	1 oz.	96
Malt-O-Meal, dry, quick cooking	1 oz.	100
(Pillsbury)	⅔ cup	200
FAT, COOKING (*Crisco; Fluffo*)	1 T.	110
FENNEL SEED (French's)	1 tsp.	8
FIG:		
Small	1½" fig	30
Canned, regular pack (Del Monte) whole, solids & liq.	½ cup	114
Canned, dietetic pack (Featherweight) Kadota, water pack, solids & liq.	½ cup	60
Dried, chopped	½ cup	235
FIG JUICE, *RealFig*	½ cup	61
FIGURINES (Pillsbury) all flavors	1 bar	138
FILBERT, shelled	1 oz.	180
FISH AU GRATIN, frozen (Mrs. Paul's)	5-oz. serving	248
FISH CAKE, frozen (Mrs. Paul's):		
Breaded & fried	2-oz. cake	105
Thins, breaded & fried	½ of 10-oz. pkg.	395
FISH & CHIPS, frozen:		
(Mrs. Paul's)	½ of 14-oz. pkg.	366
(Swanson) TV Brand	10¼-oz. dinner	450
(Swanson) TV Brand	5-oz. entree	290
(Van de Kamp's) batter dipped, french fried	8-oz. serving	500

Food and Description	Measure or Quantity	Calories
FISH DINNER, frozen:		
(Banquet)	8¾-oz. dinner	382
(Morton)	9-oz. dinner	253
(Van de Kamp's) batter dipped, french fried	11-oz. dinner	540
FISH FILLET, frozen:		
(Mrs. Paul's):		
Batter fried	2¼-oz. piece	142
Breaded & fried	4-oz. serving	227
Buttered	2½-oz. piece	155
Light batter, miniature	3-oz. serving	154
Parmesan	5-oz. piece	230
(Van de Kamp's):		
Batter dipped, french fried	3-oz. piece	220
Country seasoned	2.4-oz. piece	180
FISH FILLET DINNER (Van de Kamp's) batter dipped, french fried	12-oz. dinner	300
FISH KABOBS, frozen:		
(Mrs. Paul's) light batter	⅓ pkg.	200
(Van de Kamp's):		
Batter dipped, french fried	.4-oz. piece	26
Country seasoned	.4-oz. piece	29
FISH STICK, frozen:		
(Mrs. Paul's):		
Batter fried	1 stick	55
Breaded & fried	1 stick	43
(Van de Kamp's) batter dipped, french fried	1-oz. piece	62
FIT 'N FROSTY (Alba '77):		
Chocolate or marshmallow flavor	1 envelope	70
Strawberry	1 envelope	74
Vanilla	1 envelope	69
FIVE ALIVE (Snow Crop)	6 fl. oz.	85
FLAN, chilled (Breakstone)	5-oz. container	185
FLOUNDER:		
Baked	4 oz.	229
Frozen:		
(Mrs. Paul's) fillets, breaded & fried	2-oz. fillet	137
(Mrs. Paul's) with lemon butter	4¼-oz. serving	154
(Weight Watchers)	8½-oz. meal	169
(Weight Watchers)	16-oz. meal	261
FLOUR:		
(Aunt Jemima) self-rising	¼ cup	109

Food and Description	Measure or Quantity	Calories
Ballard, self-rising	¼ cup	95
Bisquick (Betty Crocker)	¼ cup	120
(Featherweight) gluton	¼ cup	105
(Featherweight) soy bean	¼ cup	117
Gold Medal (Betty Crocker)		
all-purpose of high protein	¼ cup	100
La Pina	¼ cup	100
Pillsbury's Best:		
All-purpose	¼ cup	100
Rye, medium	¼ cup	105
Sauce & gravy	2 T.	50
Self-rising	¼ cup	95
Presto, self-rising	¼ cup	98
Swans Down, cake	¼ cup	100
Wondra	¼ cup	100
FOOD STICKS (Pillsbury) all flavors	1 stick	45
FRANKEN°BERRY, cereal	1 cup	110
FRANKFURTER:		
(Armour Star) all meat	1.6-oz. frankfurter	110
(Eckrich):		
Beef or meat	1.6-oz. frankfurter	150
Beef or meat, jumbo	2-oz. frankfurter	190
Meat	1.2-oz. frankfurter	120
(Hormel):		
Beef	1.6-oz. frankfurter	139
Range Brand, *Wrangler,* smoked	1 frankfurter	160
(Hygrade):		
Beef, *Ball Park*	2-oz. frankfurter	169
All meat	1.6-oz. frankfurter	147
(Oscar Mayer):		
Beef	1.6-oz. frankfurter	145
Little Wiener	2″ frankfurter	31
Wiener	1.6-oz. frankfurter	145
Wiener, with cheese	1.6-oz. frankfurter	146
(Swift)	1.6-oz. frankfurter	150
(Vienna) beef	1.5-oz. frankfurter	132
(Wilson):		
Regular	1.6-oz. frankfurter	136
Skinless	1.6-oz. frankfurter	140
FRANKS-N-BLANKETS (Durkee)	1 piece	45
FRENCH TOAST, frozen:		
(Aunt Jemima):		
Regular	1½-oz. slice	85
Cinnamon swirl	1 slice	96

Food and Description	Measure or Quantity	Calories
(Eggo)	1 slice	80
(Swanson) with sausage	4½-oz. breakfast	300
FRITTERS, frozen (Mrs. Paul's):		
Apple	2-oz. fritter	117
Clam	½ of pkg.	260
Crab	½ of pkg.	250
Shrimp	½ of pkg.	240
Tuna	½ of pkg.	270
FROOT LOOPS, cereal (Kellogg's)	1 cup	110
FROSTED RICE, cereal (Kellogg's)	1 cup	110
FROZEN DESSERT, dietetic (SugarLo) all flavors	¼ pt.	135
FRUIT BITS, dried (Sun-Maid)	2-oz. serving	150
FRUIT BRUTE, cereal (General Mills)	1 cup	110
FRUIT COCKTAIL:		
Canned, regular pack, solids & liq.		
(Del Monte) regular and chunky	½ cup	95
(Libby's)	½ cup	101
(Stokely-Van Camp)	½ cup	95
Canned, dietetic pack, solids & liq.		
(Del Monte) *Lite*	½ cup	52
(Diet Delight):		
Syrup pack	½ cup	60
Water pack	½ cup	40
(Featherweight):		
Juice pack	½ cup	50
Water pack	½ cup	40
(Libby's) water pack	½ cup	40
(S&W) *Nutradiet:*		
Juice pack	½ cup	50
Water pack	½ cup	40
(Tillie Lewis) *Tasti-Diet*	½ cup	54
*FRUIT COUNTRY (Comstock):		
Apple	¼ of pkg.	160
Blueberry	¼ of pkg.	160
Cherry	¼ of pkg.	180
Peach	¼ of pkg.	130
FRUIT CUP (Del Monte):		
Mixed fruits	5-oz. container	110
Peaches, diced	5-oz. container	116
FRUIT, MIXED:		
Canned (Del Monte) *Lite*	½ cup	57
Frozen (Birds Eye)	5-oz. serving	143

Food and Description	Measure or Quantity	Calories
FRUIT PUNCH:		
Canned:		
(Ann Page) tropical	1 cup	122
(Hi-C)	6 fl. oz.	93
(Lincoln) party	6 fl. oz.	104
Chilled:		
Five Alive (Snow Crop)	6 fl. oz.	87
(Minute Maid)	6 fl. oz.	93
*Frozen, *Five Alive* (Snow Crop)	6 fl. oz.	87
*Mix (Hi-C)	6 fl. oz.	72
FRUIT ROLL, frozen (La Choy)	.5-oz. roll	38
FRUIT SALAD:		
Canned, regular pack:		
(Del Monte) fruits for salad	½ cup	94
(Del Monte) tropical	½ cup	107
(Libby's)	½ cup	89
Canned, dietetic pack:		
(Diet Delight)	½ cup	68
(Featherweight):		
Juice pack	½ cup	50
Water pack	½ cup	40
(S&W) *Nutradiet:*		
Juice pack	½ cup	60
Water pack	½ cup	35
FUDGSICLE (Popsicle Industries)	2½-fl.-oz. bar	100

G

Food and Description	Measure or Quantity	Calories
GARLIC:		
Flakes (Gilroy)	1 tsp.	5
Powder (French's)	1 tsp.	5
Spread (Lawry's)	1 T.	79
GAZPACHO SOUP (Crosse & Blackwell)	6½-oz. serving	30
GELFILTE FISH:		
(Manischewitz) 1-lb. jar	2.2-oz. piece	60
(Mother's) 1-lb. jar	2.7-oz. piece	37
***GELATIN DESSERT MIX:**		
Regular:		
(Jell-O)	½ cup	80
(Royal)	½ cup	82
Dietetic:		
(Dia-Mel) *Gel-a-Thin*	4-oz. serving	10
(D-Zerta)	½ cup	8
(Estee) all flavors	½ cup	40

Food and Description	Measure or Quantity	Calories
(Featherweight) artificially sweetened	½ cup	10
(Louis Sherry) *Shimmer*	½ cup	10
GELATIN DRINK (Knox) orange	1 envelope	70
GERMAN STYLE DINNER (Swanson) TV Brand	11¾-oz. dinner	430
GIN, SLOE:		
(Bols)	1 fl. oz.	85
(DeKuyper)	1 fl. oz.	70
(Hiram Walker)	1 fl. oz.	68
(Mr. Boston)	1 fl. oz.	68
GIN & TONIC, canned (Party Tyme) 10% alcohol	2 fl. oz.	55
GINGER, powder (French's)	1 tsp.	6
*****GINGERBREAD MIX:**		
(Betty Crocker)	⅑ of cake	210
(Dromedary)	2" x 2" square	100
(Pillsbury)	3" square	190
GOLDEN GRAHAMS, cereal (General Mills)	1 cup	110
GOOBER GRAPE (Smucker's)	1 oz.	125
GOOD HUMOR:		
Chocolate eclair	3-oz. piece	220
Sandwich	2½-oz. piece	200
Strawberry shortcake	3-oz. piece	200
Vanilla, chocolate coated	3-oz. piece	170
Whammy, assorted	1.6-oz. piece	100
Whammy, chip crunch	1.6-oz. piece	110
Whammy, ice assorted	1.5-oz. piece	50
GOOD N' PUDDIN (Popsicle Industries) all flavors	2¼-fl.-oz. bar	170
GOOSE, roasted, meat & skin	4 oz.	500
GRAHAM CRAKOS, cereal	¾ cup	110
GRANOLA BARS, *Nature Valley:*		
Almond, cinnamon or oats'n honey	1 bar	110
Coconut or peanut	1 bar	120
GRANOLA CEREAL:		
Heartland:		
Coconut	¼ cup	130
Plain or raisin	¼ cup	120
Puffs, regular or cinnamon spice	½ cup	120
Nature Valley:		
Cinnamon & raisin	⅓ cup	130
Coconut & honey	⅓ cup	150

Food and Description	Measure or Quantity	Calories
Fruit & nut	⅓ cup	130
Toasted oat	⅓ cup	130
Sun Country:		
With almonds	½ cup	250
With raisins	½ cup	250
Vita-Crunch:		
Regular	½ cup	295
Date	½ cup	284
Raisin	½ cup	289
GRANOLA CLUSTERS, *Nature Valley:*		
Almond or raisin	1 roll	140
Caramel	1 roll	150
GRAPE:		
American type (slipskin)	3½" x 3" bunch	43
Canned, dietetic (Featherweight) light, seedless, water pack	½ cup	60
GRAPE DRINK:		
Canned:		
(Hi-C)	6 fl. oz.	89
(Lincoln)	6 fl. oz.	96
*Mix (Hi-C)	6 fl. oz.	68
GRAPEFRUIT:		
Pink & red:		
Seeded type	½ med. grapefruit	46
Seedless type	½ med. grapefruit	49
White:		
Seeded type	½ med. grapefruit	44
Seedless type	½ med. grapefruit	46
Canned, regular pack (Del Monte) in syrup	½ cup	74
Canned, dietetic pack, solids & liq.:		
(Del Monte) sections	½ cup	46
(Diet Delight) sections	½ cup	46
(Featherweight) sections, juice pack	½ cup	40
(S&W) *Nutradiet*, sections	½ cup	40
(Tillie Lewis) *Tasti-Diet*	½ cup	44
GRAPEFRUIT DRINK, canned:		
(Ann Page) natural	6 fl. oz.	83
(Lincoln)	6 fl. oz.	104
GRAPEFRUIT JUICE:		
Fresh, pink, red or white	½ cup	48
Canned, sweetened:		
(Del Monte)	6 fl. oz.	89

Food and Description	Measure or Quantity	Calories
(Stokely-Van Camp)	½ cup	67
Canned, unsweetened:		
(Del Monte)	6 fl. oz.	72
(Ocean Spray)	6 fl. oz.	64
Chilled (Minute Maid)	6 fl. oz.	75
GRAPEFRUIT JUICE COCKTAIL, canned (Ocean Spray) pink	6 fl. oz.	84
GRAPEFRUIT-ORANGE JUICE COCKTAIL, canned, *Musselman's*	6 fl. oz.	67
GRAPE JAM (Smucker's)	1 T.	53
GRAPE JELLY:		
Sweetened (Smucker's)	1 T.	53
Dietetic:		
(Dia-Mel)	1 T.	6
(Diet Delight)	1 T.	13
(Featherweight)	1 T.	16
(Featherweight) artificially sweetened	1 T.	6
(S&W) *Nutradiet*, concord	1 T.	12
(Tillie Lewis) *Tasti-Diet*	1 T.	11
GRAPE JUICE:		
Canned, unsweetened (Seneca Foods) added Vitamin C	6 fl. oz.	118
*Frozen (Minute Maid) unsweetened	6 fl. oz.	99
GRAPE NUTS, cereal:		
Flakes	¾ cup	108
Nuggets	¾ cup	107
GRAPE SPREAD, dietetic:		
(Estee)	1 T.	18
(Smucker's)	1 T.	24
GRAVY, canned:		
Au jus (Franco-American)	2-oz. serving	10
Beef:		
(Ann Page)	2-oz. serving	22
(Franco-American)	2-oz. serving	30
Brown:		
(Dawn Fresh) with mushroom broth	2-oz. serving	18
(Franco-American) with onion	2-oz. serving	25
(La Choy)	5-oz. can	417
Ready Gravy	¼ cup	43
Chicken:		
(Franco-American)	2-oz. serving	50
(Franco-American) giblet	2-oz. serving	35

Food and Description	Measure or Quantity	Calories
Mushroom (Franco-American)	2-oz. serving	35
Turkey (Franco-American)	2-oz. serving	30
GRAVYMASTER	1 tsp.	12
GRAVY WITH MEAT OR TURKEY:		
Canned (Morton House):		
Sliced beef	6¼-oz. serving	190
Sliced pork	6¼-oz. serving	190
Sliced turkey	6¼-oz. serving	140
Frozen:		
(Banquet):		
Giblet gravy & sliced turkey	5-oz. bag	98
Sliced beef	2-lb. pkg.	782
(Green Giant) *Toast Topper:*		
Sliced beef	5-oz. serving	122
Sliced turkey	5-oz. serving	92
(Swanson) sliced beef with whipped potatoes	8-oz. entree	190
GRAVY MIX:		
Regular:		
Au jus:		
*(Durkee)	½ cup	15
(Durkee) *Roastin' Bag*	1-oz. pkg.	64
*(French's) *Gravy Makins*	½ cup	16
Brown:		
*(Durkee):		
Regular	½ cup	29
With mushrooms	½ cup	29
With onions	½ cup	33
*(Ehler's)	½ cup	44
*(French's) *Gravy Makins*	½ cup	40
*(Pillsbury)	½ cup	30
*(Spatini)	1-oz. serving	10
Chicken:		
(Durkee):		
*Regular	½ cup	43
*Creamy	½ cup	78
Roastin Bag	1½-oz. pkg.	122
Roastin Bag, creamy	2-oz. pkg.	242
*(French's) *Gravy Makins*	½ cup	50
*(Pillsbury)	½ cup	30
Home style:		
*(Durkee)	½ cup	35
*(French's) *Gravy Makins*	½ cup	50
*(Pillsbury)	½ cup	30
Meatloaf (Durkee) *Roastin' Bag*	1½-oz. pkg.	129

Food and Description	Measure or Quantity	Calories
Mushroom:		
*(Durkee)	½ cup	30
*(French's) *Gravy Makins*	½ cup	40
Onion:		
*(Durkee)	½ cup	42
*(French's) *Gravy Makins*	½ cup	50
Pork:		
*(Durkee)	½ cup	35
*(French's) *Gravy Makins*	½ cup	40
*Swiss steak (Durkee)	½ cup	23
Turkey:		
*(Durkee)	½ cup	23
*(French's) *Gravy Makins*	½ cup	50
*Dietetic (Weight Watchers):		
Brown	½ cup	16
Brown, with mushrooms	½ cup	24
Brown, with onion	½ cup	26
Chicken	½ cup	20
GRENADINE (Garnier) no alcohol	1 fl. oz.	103
GUAVA	1 guava	48

H

HADDOCK:		
Fried, breaded	4" x 3" x ½" fillet	165
Frozen:		
(Banquet)	8¾-oz. dinner	419
(Mrs. Paul's):		
Breaded & fried	2-oz. fillet	114
Buttered fillets	5-oz. serving	200
(Van de Kamp's) batter dipped, french fried	2.3-oz. piece	165
(Weight Watchers)	16-oz. meal	261
Smoked	4-oz. serving	117
HALIBUT:		
Broiled	4" x 3" x ½" steak	214
Frozen (Van de Kamp's) batter dipped, french fried	1.3-oz. piece	90
HAM:		
Canned:		
(Hormel):		
Chunk	6¾-oz. serving	329
Chopped	¼ of 12-oz. can	229
EXL	4-oz. serving	128
Holiday Glaze	4 oz. serving	140
Patties	1 patty	200

Food and Description	Measure or Quantity	Calories
(Oscar Mayer) *Jubilee*, extra lean, cooked	1-oz. serving	31
(Swift)		
Hostess	3½-oz. slice	141
Premium	1¾-oz. slice	111
Deviled:		
(Hormel)	1 oz.	71
(Libby's)	1 oz.	85
(Underwood)	¼ of 4½-oz. can	97
Packaged:		
(Eckrich) cooked, sliced	1.2-oz. slice	37
(Hormel):		
Black or red peppered	.8-oz. slice	26
Chopped	1-oz. slice	61
Cooked	.8-oz. slice	26
Cooked, smoked	.8-oz. slice	28
(Oscar Mayer):		
Chopped	1-oz. slice	64
Cooked, smoked	¾-oz. slice	25
Cooked, smoked	1-oz. slice	34
Jubilee, sliced, boneless	8-oz. slice	264
Jubilee, steak, boneless, 95% fat free	2-oz. steak	69
HAMBURGER (See *McDONALD'S* and *BURGER KING*)		
HAMBURGER MIX:		
(Ann Page):		
Beef noodle	⅕ of 7-oz. pkg.	146
Chili tomato	⅕ of 8-oz. pkg.	156
Potato stroganoff	⅕ of 7-oz. pkg.	141
Hamburger Helper (General Mills):		
Beef noodle	⅕ of pkg.	320
Beef romanoff	⅕ of pkg.	340
Cheeseburger	⅕ of pkg.	360
Chili tomato	⅕ of pkg.	320
Hash	⅕ of pkg.	300
Lasagna	⅕ of pkg.	330
Pizza	⅕ of pkg.	320
Potatoes au gratin	⅕ of pkg.	320
Potatoes stroganoff	⅕ of pkg.	320
Rice oriental	⅕ of pkg.	340
Spaghetti	⅕ of pkg.	330
Stew	⅕ of pkg.	290
Make A Better Burger (Lipton) mildly seasoned or onion	1 patty	180

Food and Description	Measure or Quantity	Calories
HAMBURGER SEASONING MIX:		
*(Durkee)	1 cup	663
(French's)	1-oz. pkg.	100
HAM & BUTTER BEAN SOUP, canned (Campbell) *Chunky*	10¾-oz. can	290
HAM & CHEESE:		
(Hormel) loaf	1-oz. serving	69
(Oscar Mayer) loaf	1-oz. serving	77
HAM DINNER, frozen:		
(Banquet)	10-oz. dinner	369
(Morton)	10-oz. dinner	449
(Swanson) TV Brand	10¼-oz. dinner	380
HAM SALAD, canned (Carnation)	1½-oz. serving	78
HAM SALAD SPREAD		
(Oscar Mayer)	1 oz.	62
HAWAIIAN PUNCH:		
Canned:		
Cherry	6 fl. oz.	87
Grape	6 fl. oz.	93
Orange	6 fl. oz.	97
Red	6 fl. oz.	84
Very berry	6 fl. oz.	87
*Mix, red punch	8 fl. oz.	100
HEADCHEESE (Oscar Mayer)	1-oz. serving	54
HERRING, canned (Vita):		
Bismarck, drained	5-oz. jar	273
Cocktail, drained	8-oz. jar	342
In cream sauce	8-oz. jar	397
Marjes, drained	8-oz. jar	304
Tastee Bits, drained	8-oz. jar	361
HERRING, SMOKED, kippered	4-oz. serving	239
HICKORY NUT, shelled	1-oz. serving	191
HO-HO (Hostess)	1-oz. cake	124
HOMINY GRITS:		
Dry:		
(Albers)	1½ oz.	150
(Aunt Jemima)	3 T.	101
(Quaker):		
Regular	3 T.	101
Instant:		
Regular	.8-oz. packet	79
With imitation bacon or ham	1-oz. packet	101
With imitation cheese flavor	1-oz. packet	104
Cooked	1 cup	125

Food and Description	Measure or Quantity	Calories
HONEY, strained	1 T.	61
HONEYCOMB, cereal	1⅓ cups	113
HONEYDEW	2" x 7" wedge	31
HOPPING JOHN (Green Giant)	½ of pkg.	116
HORSERADISH:		
Raw, pared	1 oz.	25
Prepared (Gold's)	1-oz. serving	18

I

Food and Description	Measure or Quantity	Calories
ICE CREAM & FROZEN CUSTARD (See also listing by flavor or brand name or FROZEN DESSERT):		
(Dean) 10.4% fat	1 cup	336
ICE CREAM CONE, cone only (Comet):		
Regular	1 piece	20
Rolled sugar	1 piece	40
ICE CREAM CUP, cup only (Comet)	1 cup	20
ICE CREAM SANDWICH (Sealtest)	3 fl. oz.	170
ICE MILK:		
Hardened	¼ pt.	100
Soft-serve	¼ pt.	133
(Dean) *Count Calorie*	¼ pt.	99
(Meadow Gold) vanilla, 4% fat	¼ pt.	95
ITALIAN DINNER, frozen (Banquet)	11-oz. dinner	456

J

Food and Description	Measure or Quantity	Calories
JAM, sweetened (Ann Page) all flavors	1 tsp.	19
JELLY, sweetened (See also individual flavors):		
(Ann Page) all flavors	1 T.	18
(Crosse & Blackwell) all flavors	1 T.	51
JERUSALEM ARTICHOKE, pared	4 oz.	75
JOHANNISBERG RIESLING:		
(Deinhard)	3 fl. oz.	72
(Inglenook)	3 fl. oz.	61
JUNIORS (Tastykake):		
Chocolate	2¾-oz. pkg.	307

Food and Description	Measure or Quantity	Calories
Coconut	2¾-oz. pkg.	330
Koffee Kake	2½-oz. pkg.	313
Lemon	2¾-oz. pkg.	297

K

Food and Description	Measure or Quantity	Calories
KABOOM, cereal (General Mills)	1 cup	110
KALE:		
Boiled, leaves only	4 oz.	44
Frozen:		
(Birds Eye) chopped	⅓ of pkg.	30
(McKenzie) chopped	⅓ of pkg.	32
(Seabrook Farms) chopped	⅓ of pkg.	32
KANDY KAKES (Tastykake):		
Chocolate	1.3-oz. pkg.	60
Peanut butter	1.3-oz. pkg.	190
KARO SYRUP (See SYRUP)		
KEFIR (Alta-Dena Dairy):		
Plain	1 cup	180
Flavored	1 cup	190
KIDNEY:		
Beef, braised	4 oz.	286
Calf, raw	4 oz.	128
Lamb, raw	4 oz.	119
KIELBASA:		
(Eckrich) skinless	2-oz. serving	190
(Hormel) Kolbase	2-oz. serving	245
(Vienna)	2-oz. serving	165
KING VITAMAN, cereal	¾ cup	120
KIRSCH, liqueur (Garnier)	1 fl. oz.	83
KIX, cereal	1½ cups	110
KNOCKWURST	1 oz.	79
KOOL-AID (General Foods):		
Unsweetened	8 fl. oz.	93
Sweetened:		
All flavors except tropical punch	8 fl. oz.	93
Tropical punch	8 fl. oz.	98
KUMQUAT, flesh & skin	5 oz.	74

L

Food and Description	Measure or Quantity	Calories
LAMB:		
Leg:		
Roasted, lean & fat	3 oz.	237
Roasted, lean only	3 oz.	158

Food and Description	Measure or Quantity	Calories
Loin, one 5-oz. chop (weighed with bone before cooking) will give you:		
Lean & fat	2.8 oz.	280
Lean only	2.3 oz.	122
Rib, one 5-oz. chop (weighed with bone before cooking) will give you:		
Lean & fat	2.9 oz.	334
Lean only	2 oz.	118
Shoulder:		
Roasted, lean & fat	3 oz.	287
Roasted, lean only	3 oz.	174
LASAGNA:		
Canned:		
(Hormel) *Short Orders*	7½-oz. can	260
(Nalley's)	8-oz. serving	239
Frozen:		
(Green Giant):		
With meat sauce, *Bake 'n Serve*	7-oz. serving	295
With meat sauce, boil-in-bag	9-oz. bag	294
(Hormel) beef	10-oz. serving	371
(Stouffer's)	10½-oz. serving	380
(Swanson):		
Hungry Man	17¾-oz. dinner	790
Hungry Man, with meat	12¾-oz. entree	540
With meat in tomato sauce	11¾-oz. entree	450
TV brand	13-oz. dinner	390
LEEKS	4 oz.	59
LEMON:		
Whole	2⅛" lemon	22
Peeled	2⅛" lemon	20
LEMONADE:		
Canned:		
Country Time	6 fl. oz.	89
(Hi-C)	6 fl. oz.	68
Chilled (Minute Maid) regular or pink	6 fl. oz.	79
*Frozen:		
Country Time, regular or pink	6 fl. oz.	68
Minute Maid	6 fl. oz.	74
(Sunkist) regular or pink	6 fl. oz.	81
*Mix:		
Country Time, regular or pink	6 fl. oz.	68
(Hi-C)	6 fl. oz.	76

Food and Description	Measure or Quantity	Calories
Kool Aid, sweetened, regular or pink	6 fl. oz.	75
Kool Aid, unsweetened, regular or pink	6 fl. oz.	67
Lemon Tree (Lipton)	6 fl. oz.	68
(Minute Maid) regular or pink	6 fl. oz.	80
LEMON EXTRACT (Virginia Dare)	1 tsp.	22
LEMON JUICE:		
Canned, *ReaLemon*	1 T.	3
*Frozen (Minute Maid) unsweetened	1 fl. oz.	7
*LEMON-LIMEADE, mix (Minute Maid)	6 fl. oz.	80
LEMON PEEL, candied	1 oz.	90
LEMON-PEPPER SEASONING (French's)	1 tsp.	6
LENTIL SOUP:		
(Crosse & Blackwell) with ham	6½-oz. serving	80
(Progresso)	1 cup	150
LETTUCE:		
Bibb or Boston	4″ head	23
Cos or Romaine, shredded or broken into pieces	½ cup	4
Grand Rapids, Salad Bowl or Simpson	2 large leaves	9
Iceberg, New York or Great Lakes	¼ of 4¾″ head	15
LIEBFRAUMILCH WINE:		
(Anheuser)	3 fl. oz.	63
(Deinhard)	3 fl. oz.	60
(Julius Kayser) Glockenspiel	3 fl. oz.	57
LIFE cereal (Quaker) regular or cinnamon	⅔ cup	105
LIME, peeled	2″ dia.	15
*LIMEADE, frozen (Minute Maid)	6 fl. oz.	75
LIME ICE, home recipe	4 oz.	88
LIME JUICE, *ReaLime*	1 T.	2
LINGUINI IN CLAM SAUCE, frozen:		
(Ronzoni)	4-oz. serving	120
(Stouffer's)	5¼-oz. serving	142
LIVER:		
Beef:		
Fried	6½″ x 2⅜″ x ⅜″ slice	195
Cooked (Swift)	3.2-oz. serving	141

Food and Description	Measure or Quantity	Calories
Calf, fried	6½" x 2⅜" x ⅜" slice	222
Chicken, simmered	2" x 2" x ⅝" liver	41
LIVERWURST SPREAD		
(Underwood)	1-oz. serving	92
LOBSTER:		
Cooked, meat only	1 cup	138
Canned, meat only	4-oz. serving	108
Frozen, South African lobster tail:		
3 in 8-oz. pkg.	1 piece	87
4 in 8-oz. pkg.	1 piece	65
5 in 8-oz. pkg.	1 piece	51
LOBSTER NEWBURG	1 cup	485
LOBSTER PASTE, canned	1-oz. serving	51
LOBSTER SALAD	4-oz. serving	125
LOBSTER SOUP, cream of (Crosse & Blackwell)	6½-oz. serving	92
LOG CABIN SYRUP (See SYRUP)		
LOQUAT, fresh, flesh only	2 oz.	27
LUCKY CHARMS, cereal (General Mills)	1 cup	110
LUNCHEON MEAT (See also individual listings, e.g., BOLOGNA, HAM, etc.)		
All meat (Oscar Mayer)	1-oz. slice	98
Banquet loaf (Eckrich)	1-oz. slice	75
Bar-B-Que loaf (Oscar Mayer) 90% fat free	1-oz. slice	49
BBQ loaf (Hormel)	1-oz. slice	50
Beef honey roll sausage (Oscar Mayer) 90% fat free	.8-oz. slice	40
Beef, jellied (Hormel) loaf	1.2-oz. slice	35
Buffet loaf (Hormel)	1-oz. slice	50
Gourmet loaf (Eckrich)	1-oz. slice	32
Ham & cheese (See HAM & CHEESE)		
Ham roll sausage (Oscar Mayer)	.8-oz. slice	35
Ham roll sausage (Oscar Mayer)	1-oz. slice	43
Honey loaf:		
(Eckrich)	1-oz. slice	40
(Hormel)	1-oz. slice	47
(Oscar Mayer) 95% fat free	1-oz. slice	35
Liver cheese (Oscar Mayer)	1.3-oz. slice	114
Liver loaf (Hormel)	1-oz. slice	81
Luxury loaf (Oscar Mayer) 95% fat free	1-oz. slice	39

Food and Description	Measure or Quantity	Calories
Meat loaf	1-oz. serving	57
New England brand sliced sausage:		
(Hormel)	1-oz. slice	49
(Oscar Mayer) 92% fat free	.5-oz. slice	22
(Oscar Mayer) 92% fat free	.8-oz. slice	34
Old fashioned loaf:		
(Eckrich)	1-oz. slice	75
(Oscar Mayer)	1-oz. slice	65
Olive loaf:		
(Hormel)	1-oz. slice	59
(Oscar Mayer)	1-oz. slice	65
Peppered beef (Vienna)	1-oz. serving	50
Peppered loaf:		
(Hormel)	1-oz. serving	72
(Oscar Mayer) 93% fat free	1-oz. slice	42
Pickle loaf:		
(Eckrich)	1-oz. slice	85
(Hormel)	1-oz. slice	59
Pickle & pimento (Oscar Mayer)	1-oz. slice	65
Picnic loaf (Oscar Mayer)	1-oz. slice	64
Spiced (Hormel)	1-oz. serving	77

M

MACADAMIA NUT		
(Royal Hawaiian)	1 oz.	197
MACARONI, cooked:		
8-10 minutes, firm	1 cup	192
14-20 minutes, tender	1 cup	155
MACARONI & BEEF:		
Canned, in tomato sauce:		
(Franco-American) *Beefy Mac*	7½-oz. can	230
(Nalley's)	8-oz. serving	236
Frozen:		
(Banquet)	12-oz. dinner	394
(Banquet) buffet	2-lb. pkg.	1000
(Green Giant)	9-oz. entree	233
(Stouffer's)	11½-oz. pkg.	384
(Swanson) TV Brand	12-oz. dinner	400
MACARONI & CHEESE:		
Canned:		
(Franco-American)	7⅜-oz. serving	180
(Franco-American) elbow	7⅜-oz. serving	105
(Hormel) *Short Orders*	7½-oz. can	170

Food and Description	Measure or Quantity	Calories
Frozen:		
(Banquet):		
Buffet	2-lb. pkg.	1027
Dinner	12-oz. dinner	326
(Green Giant):		
Cooking bag	9-oz. entree	304
Oven bake	6-oz. serving	216
(Morton)	8-oz. casserole	227
(Stouffer's)	12-oz. pkg.	502
(Swanson):		
Regular	12-oz. entree	420
TV Brand	12½-oz. dinner	390
(Van de Kamp's)	10-oz. pkg.	300
Mix:		
(Ann Page) dinner	¼ of 7¼-oz. pkg.	189
(Golden Grain) deluxe	¼ of 7¼-oz. pkg.	202
*(Pennsylvania Dutch Brand)	½ cup	160
*(Prince)	¾ cup	268
MACARONI & CHEESE PIE, frozen (Swanson)	7-oz. pie	230
MACARONI DINNER, frozen (Weight Watchers) ziti	13-oz. meal	363
MACARONI SALAD, canned (Nalley's)	4-oz. serving	206
MACKEREL, Atlantic, broiled, with fat	8½" x 2½" x ½" fillet	248
MADEIRA WINE (Leacock)	3 fl. oz.	120
MAI TAI COCKTAIL:		
Canned:		
(Lemon Hart) 48 proof	3 fl. oz.	180
(Mr. Boston) 12½% alcohol	3 fl. oz.	111
(National Distillers) *Duet* 12½% alcohol	8-fl.-oz. can	288
(Party Tyme) 12½% alcohol	2 fl. oz.	65
Mix:		
Dry:		
(Bar-Tender's; Holland House)	1 serving	69
(Party Tyme)	½-oz. serving	50
Liquid, canned (Holland House)	1½ fl. oz.	50
MALTED MILK MIX (Carnation)		
Chocolate	3 heaping tsps.	85
Natural	3 heaping tsps.	90
MALT LIQUOR, *Champale,* regular	12 fl. oz.	179

Food and Description	Measure or Quantity	Calories
MANDARIN ORANGE (See TANGERINE)		
MANGO, fresh	1 med. mango	88
MANHATTAN COCKTAIL:		
Canned:		
(Hiram Walker) 55 proof	3 fl. oz.	147
(Mr. Boston) 20% alcohol	3 fl. oz.	123
Mix, dry (Bar-Tender's)	1 serving	24
Mix, liquid, canned (Holland House)	1½ fl. oz.	14
MAPLE SYRUP (See SYRUP, Maple)		
MARGARINE:		
Regular	1 pat (1" x 1.3" x 1", 5 grams)	36
(Parkay) regular, soft or squeeze	1 T.	101
MARGARINE, IMITATION or DIETETIC:		
(Parkay)	1 T.	55
(Weight Watchers)	1 T.	50
MARGARINE, WHIPPED (Blue Bonnet; Miracle; Parkay)	1 T.	67
MARGARITA COCKTAIL:		
Canned:		
(Mr. Boston):		
Regular, 12½% alcohol	3 fl. oz.	105
Strawberry, 12½% alcohol	3 fl. oz.	138
(National Distillers) *Duet*, 12½% alcohol	8-fl.-oz. can	248
Mix:		
Dry:		
(Bar-Tender's)	1 serving	70
(Party Tyme)	½-oz. serving	50
Liquid:		
(Holland House)	1½ fl. oz.	58
(Party Tyme)	2 fl. oz.	63
MARINADE MIX:		
Chicken (Adolph's)	1-oz. packet	64
Meat:		
(Adolph's)	.8-oz. pkg.	38
(Durkee)	1-oz. pkg.	47
(French's)	1-oz. pkg.	80
MARJORAM (French's)	1 tsp.	4
MARMALADE:		
Sweetened:		
(Ann Page)	1 T.	49

Food and Description	Measure or Quantity	Calories
(Keiller)	1 T.	60
(Smucker's)	1 T.	53
Dietetic:		
(Dia-Mel)	1 T.	6
(Featherweight)	1 T.	16
(Louis Sherry)	1 T.	6
(Smucker's) imitation	1 T.	24
(S&W) *Nutradiet*	1 T.	12
(Tillie Lewis) *Tasti-Diet*	1 T.	12
MARSHMALLOW FLUFF	1 heaping tsp.	59
MARTINI COCKTAIL:		
Gin, canned:		
(Hiram Walker) 67.5 proof	3 fl. oz.	168
(Mr. Boston) extra dry, 20% alcohol	3 fl. oz.	99
Gin, mix, liquid (Holland House)	2 fl. oz.	20
Vodka, canned:		
(Hiram Walker) 60 proof	3 fl. oz.	147
(Mr. Boston) 20% alcohol	3 fl. oz.	108
MASA HARINA (Quaker)	⅓ cup	137
MASA TRIGO (Quaker)	⅓ cup	149
MATZO (Horowitz Margareten)	1 matzo	120
MAYONNAISE:		
Regular:		
(Ann Page)	1 T.	105
Hellmann's (Best Foods)	1 T.	103
Imitation or dietetic:		
(Dia-Mel)	1 T.	105
(Diet Delight) imitation, *Mayo-Lite*	1 T.	26
(Featherweight) imitation, *Soyamaise*	1 T.	100
(Tillie Lewis) imitation *Tasti-Diet*	1 T.	25
(Weight Watcher) imitation	1 T.	40
MAYPO, cereal:		
30-second	¼ cup	89
Vermont-style	¼ cup	121
McDONALD'S:		
Big Mac	1 hamburger	541
Cheeseburger	1 cheeseburger	306
Cookies, *McDonaldland*	1 package	294
Egg McMuffin	1 serving	352
English muffin, buttered	1 muffin	186
Filet-O-Fish sandwich	1 sandwich	402

Food and Description	Measure or Quantity	Calories
French fries	1 regular order	211
Hamburger	1 hamburger	257
Hot cakes with butter & syrup	1 serving	471
Pie:		
Apple	1 pie	300
Cherry	1 pie	298
Quarter Pounder	1 hamburger	418
Quarter Pounder with cheese..	1 hamburger	514
Sausage, pork	1 serving	184
Scrambled eggs	1 serving	161
Shake:		
Chocolate	1 serving	363
Strawberry	1 serving	347
Vanilla	1 serving	322
MEATBALL DINNER or ENTREE frozen (Swanson) with brown gravy & whipped potatoes, TV Brand	9½-oz. entree	330
MEATBALL SEASONING MIX:		
*(Durkee) Italian style	1 cup	619
(French's)	1½-oz. pkg.	140
***MEATBALL SOUP, canned** (Campbell) condensed, alphabet	10-oz. serving	140
MEATBALL STEW, canned:		
Dinty Moore	7½-oz. serving	245
(Libby's)	12-oz. serving	281
(Morton House)	8-oz. serving	290
(Nalley's)	8-oz. serving	261
MEATBALLS, SWEDISH, frozen (Stouffer's) with noodles	11-oz. pkg.	473
MEAT LOAF DINNER, frozen:		
(Banquet):		
Regular	11-oz. dinner	412
Man-Pleaser	19-oz. dinner	916
(Morton) *Country Table*	15-oz. dinner	477
(Swanson):		
TV Brand	10¾-oz. dinner	530
TV Brand, with tomato sauce and whipped potatoes	9-oz. entree	330
MEAT LOAF SEASONING MIX:		
(Contadina)	3¾-oz. pkg.	363
(French's)	1½-oz. pkg.	160
MEAT, POTTED (Libby's)	1-oz. serving	57
MEAT TENDERIZER:		
(Adolph's)	1 tsp.	2
(French's)	1 tsp.	2

Food and Description	Measure or Quantity	Calories
MELBA TOAST, salted (Old London):		
Garlic, onion or white rounds	1 piece	10
Pumpernickel, rye, wheat or white	1 piece	17
Sesame, flat	1 piece	18
Sesame, round	1 piece	11
MELON BALL, in syrup, frozen	½ cup	72
MEXICAN DINNER, frozen:		
(Banquet) combination	12-oz. dinner	571
(Swanson) TV Brand, combination	16-oz. dinner	700
(Van de Kamp's) combination	11-oz. dinner	420
MILK, CONDENSED, *Dime Brand*; *Eagle Brand*; *Magnolia Brand*	1 T.	60
*MILK, DRY, non-fat, instant (Alba; Carnation; Pet)	1 cup	80
MILK, EVAPORATED:		
Regular:		
(Carnation)	4 fl. oz.	42
(Pet)	1 fl. oz.	43
Filled:		
Dairymate	½ cup	150
(Pet)	½ cup	150
Low fat (Carnation)	1 fl. oz.	28
Skimmed:		
(Carnation)	1 fl. oz.	24
Pet 99	1 fl. oz.	25
MILK, FRESH:		
(Dean; Sealtest) whole, 3.5% fat	1 cup	151
(Sealtest) extra rich, Vitamin D	1 cup	170
Skim:		
(Dean) 2% fat	1 cup	133
(Meadow Gold) Vitamins A & D	1 cup	90
(Meadow Gold) *Viva*, 2% fat, Vitamins A & D	1 cup	130
(Sealtest)	1 cup	79
Buttermilk:		
(Dean)	1 cup	95
(Sealtest) protein fortified	1 cup	110
Chocolate:		
(Dean) with whole milk	1 cup	212
(Dean) with skim milk, 1% fat	1 cup	166
(Sealtest) Vitamin D	1 cup	190
MILK, GOAT, whole	1 cup	163

Food and Description	Measure or Quantity	Calories
MILK, HUMAN	1 oz.	22
MINESTRONE SOUP:		
*(Ann Page)	1 cup	82
(Campbell):		
Chunky	19-oz. can	280
*Condensed	10-oz. serving	90
(Crosse & Blackwell)	6½-oz. serving	90
MINI-WHEATS, cereal	1 biscuit	27
MINT LEAVES	½ oz.	4
MOLASSES:		
Barbados	1 T.	51
Blackstrap	1 T.	40
Dark (Brer Rabbit)	1 T.	33
Light	1 T.	48
Medium	1 T.	44
Unsulphured (Grandma's)	1 T.	60
MORTADELLA, sausage	1 oz.	89
MOSELLE WINE (Great Western)	3 fl. oz.	72
MOST, cereal	¾ cup	110
MUFFIN:		
Blueberry (Morton) frozen:		
Regular	1.6-oz. muffin	125
Rounds	1.5-oz. muffin	115
Bran (Arnold) *Orowheat*	2.3-oz. muffin	160
Corn:		
(Morton) frozen:		
Regular	1.7-oz. muffin	129
Rounds	1.5-oz. muffin	127
(Thomas')	2-oz. muffin	184
English:		
(Arnold) extra crisp	2.3-oz. muffin	150
Home Pride	2-oz. muffin	136
Home Pride, wheat	2-oz. muffin	141
(Pepperidge Farm)	1 muffin	140
(Pepperidge Farm) cinnamon raisin	1 muffin	150
(Thomas')	2-oz. muffin	133
(Thomas') onion	2-oz. muffin	129
(Wonder)	2-oz. muffin	130
Plain	1.4-oz. muffin	118
Plain		
(Arnold) Orowheat	2.5-oz. muffin	170
(Wonder) rounds	2-oz. muffin	150
Sourdough (Wonder)	2-oz. muffin	135
MUFFIN MIX:		
Blueberry:		
*(Betty Crocker) wild	1 muffin	120

Food and Description	Measure or Quantity	Calories
(Duncan Hines)	1/12 of pkg.	99
Corn:		
*(Betty Crocker)	1 muffin	160
*(Dromedary)	1 muffin	130
*(Flako)	1 muffin	140
MUG-O-LUNCH (General Mills):		
Chicken flavored noodles & sauce	1 pouch	150
Macaroni & cheese sauce	1 pouch	230
Noodles & beef flavored sauce	1 pouch	170
Spaghetti & tomato sauce	1 pouch	160
MULLIGAN STEW, canned, *Dinty Moore, Short Orders*	7½-oz. can	230
MUSCATEL WINE (Gallo) 14% alcohol	3 fl. oz.	86
MUSHROOM:		
Raw, whole	½ lb.	62
Raw, trimmed, sliced	½ cup	10
Canned:		
(Green Giant)	2-oz. serving	12
(Shady Oaks)	4-oz. can	19
Frozen (Green Giant) whole, in butter sauce	3-oz. serving	42
MUSHROOM, CHINESE, dried	1 oz.	81
MUSHROOM SOUP:		
Canned, regular pack:		
*(Ann Page) cream of	1 cup	126
*(Campbell) condensed:		
Cream of	10-oz. serving	120
Cream of, *Soup For One*	7½-oz. can	140
Golden	10-oz. serving	110
(Crosse & Blackwell) cream of, bisque	6½-oz. serving	90
Canned, dietetic pack:		
(Campbell) cream of, low sodium	7¼-oz. can	140
*(Dia-Mel)	8-oz. serving	45
MUSHROOM SOUP MIX:		
*(Lipton):		
Beef	8-oz. serving	45
Cream of, *Cup-a-Soup*	6 fl. oz.	80
*(Nestlé) *Souptime*, cream of	6 fl. oz.	80
MUSSEL, in shell	1 lb.	153
MUSTARD:		
Powder (French's)	1 tsp.	9
Prepared:		
Brown (French's; Gulden's;		

Food and Description	Measure or Quantity	Calories
Grey Poupon)	1 tsp.	5
Horseradish (Nalley's)	1 tsp.	5
Salad, cream (French's)	1 tsp.	3
Yellow (Gulden's)	1 tsp.	5
MUSTARD GREENS, frozen:		
(Birds Eye)	⅓ of pkg.	20
(McKenzie)	⅓ of pkg.	25
(Seabrook Farms)	⅓ of pkg.	25
MUSTARD SPINACH:		
Raw	1 lb.	100
Boiled, drained, no added salt	4-oz. serving	18

N

Food and Description	Measure or Quantity	Calories
NATURAL CEREAL:		
Heartland:		
Regular	¼ cup	120
Coconut	¼ cup	130
(Quaker):		
Hot, whole wheat	⅓ cup	100
100%	¼ cup	139
100% with apple & cinnamon	¼ cup	135
100% with raisins & dates	¼ cup	134
NATURE SNACKS (Sun-Maid):		
Carob Crunch	1 oz.	150
CoCo Banana	1 oz.	140
Go-Bananas	1 oz.	280
Nuts Galore	1 oz.	170
Raisin Crunch	1 oz.	130
Rocky Road	1 oz.	160
Tahitian Treat	1 oz.	140
NECTARINE, flesh only	4 oz.	73
NEOPOLITAN CREAM PIE, frozen (Morton)	⅙ of 16-oz. pie	192
NOODLE:		
Dry (Pennsylvania Dutch Brand) broad	1 oz.	125
Cooked, 1½" strips	1 cup	200
NOODLES & BEEF:		
Canned (Hormel) *Short Orders*	7½-oz. can	230
Frozen (Banquet) buffet	2-lb. pkg.	754
NOODLE & CHICKEN:		
Canned, *Dinty Moore, Short Orders*	7½-oz. can	210
Frozen (Swanson) TV Brand	10¼-oz. dinner	390

Food and Description	*Measure or Quantity*	*Calories*
NOODLE, CHOW MEIN:		
(Chun King)	⅙ of 5-oz. can	100
(La Choy):		
Regular	½ cup	153
Wide	½ cup	149
NOODLE MIX:		
*(Betty Crocker):		
Almondine	¼ of pkg.	240
Romanoff	¼ of pkg.	230
Stroganoff	¼ of pkg.	240
Noodle Roni, parmesano	⅙ of 6-oz. pkg.	130
*(Pennsylvania Dutch Brand)		
Noodles Plus Sauce:		
Beef	½ cup	130
Butter	½ cup	150
Cheese	½ cup	150
Chicken	½ cup	150
**Side Quicks* (General Mills)		
all varieties	¼ pkg.	120
**Tuna Helper:*		
Almondine	¼ of pkg.	240
Romanoff	¼ pkg.	230
Stroganoff	¼ of pkg.	230
***NOODLE, RAMEN (La Choy)**		
canned:		
Beef	1 cup	225
Chicken	1 cup	202
Oriental	1 cup	207
NOODLE, RICE (La Choy)	1 oz.	130
NOODLE ROMANOFF, frozen		
(Stouffer's)	⅓ of pkg.	168
***NOODLE SOUP (Campbell):**		
Curly with chicken	10-oz. serving	100
& ground beef	10-oz. serving	110
NUT, MIXED:		
Dry roasted:		
(A&P)	1 oz.	179
(Flavor House)	1 oz.	172
(Planters)	1 oz.	160
Oil roasted:		
(Excel) with peanuts	1 oz.	187
(Planters) with peanuts	1 oz.	180
(Planters) without peanuts	1 oz.	180
NUTMEG (French's)	1 tsp.	11
NUT*Os (General Mills)	1 T.	35
NUTRIMATO (Mott's)	6 fl. oz.	70

Food and Description	Measure or Quantity	Calories

O

Food and Description	Measure or Quantity	Calories
OAT FLAKES, cereal (Post)	⅔ cup	107
OATMEAL:		
Dry:		
Regular:		
(H-O) old fashioned	1 T.	15
(H-O) old fashioned	½ cup	139
(Quaker) old fashioned	⅓ cup	109
(Ralston Purina)	⅓ cup	110
Instant:		
(H-O)		
Regular, boxed	1 T.	15
Regular, boxed	½ cup	129
Regular, packets	1-oz. packet	105
With bran & spice	1½-oz. packet	157
With cinnamon & spice	1⅝-oz. packet	175
With country apple & brown sugar	1.1-oz. packet	121
With maple & brown sugar flavor	1½-oz. packet	160
Sweet & mellow	1.4-oz. packet	149
(Quaker):		
Regular	1-oz. packet	105
Apple & cinnamon	1¼-oz. packet	134
Bran & raisin	1½-oz. packet	153
Cinnamon & spice	1⅝-oz. packet	176
Maple & brown sugar	1½-oz. packet	163
Raisins & spice	1½-oz. packet	159
(3-Minute Brand) *Stir'N Eat*:		
Dutch apple brown sugar	1⅛-oz. packet	120
Natural flavor	1-oz. packet	106
Quick:		
(Harvest Brand)	⅓ cup	108
(H-O)	½ cup	129
(Quaker) old fashioned	⅓ cup	109
(Ralston Purina)	⅓ cup	110
(3-Minute Brand)	⅓ cup	108
Cooked, regular	1 cup	132
OCEAN PERCH:		
Fried	4-oz. serving	257
Frozen (Banquet)	8¾-oz. dinner	434

Food and Description	Measure or Quantity	Calories
OIL, SALAD or COOKING:		
Crisco; Fleischmann's; Mazola; Puritan	1 T.	126
Golden Thistle; Mrs. Tucker's; Planters	1 T.	130
Saffola	1 T.	124
Sunlite; Wesson	1 T.	120
OKRA, frozen:		
(Birds Eye) whole	⅓ of pkg.	30
(Green Giant) gumbo	⅓ of pkg.	83
(McKenzie) cut	⅓ of pkg.	32
(Seabrook Farms) cut	⅓ of pkg.	32
(Seabrook Farms) whole	⅓ of pkg.	36
OLD FASHIONED COCKTAIL:		
Canned (Hiram Walker) 62 proof	3 fl. oz.	165
Mix, dry (Bar-Tender's)	1 serving	20
OLIVE:		
Green	4 med. or 3 extra large or 2 giant	19
Ripe, Mission	3 small or 2 large	18
ONION:		
Raw	2½" onion	38
Boiled, pearl onion	½ cup	27
Canned (Durkee) *O & C:*		
Boiled	¼ of 16-oz. jar	32
Creamed	¼ of 15½-oz. can	554
Dehydrated (Gilroy) flakes	1 tsp.	5
Frozen:		
(Birds Eye):		
Chopped	⅓ of pkg.	8
Creamed	⅓ of pkg.	100
Whole	⅓ of pkg.	40
(Green Giant) creamed	⅓ of pkg.	50
(Mrs. Paul's) french-fried rings	½ of 5-oz. pkg.	156
(Ore-Ida):		
Chopped	2 oz.	20
Onion Ringers	2-oz. serving	160
ONION BOUILLON:		
(Croydon House)	1 tsp.	11
(Herb-Ox)	1 cube	10
MBT	1 packet	16
ONION, GREEN	1 small onion	4
ONION SALAD SEASONING (French's) instant	1 T.	15

Food and Description	Measure or Quantity	Calories
ONION SOUP, canned:		
*(Campbell):		
Regular	10-oz. serving	80
Cream of, made with water	10-oz. serving	130
Cream of, made with milk & water	10-oz. serving	180
(Crosse & Blackwell)	6½-oz. serving	45
ONION SOUP MIX:		
(Ann Page)	1⅜-oz. pkg.	115
*(Lipton):		
Regular	1 cup	40
Beefy	1 cup	30
Cup-a-Soup	1 pkg.	30
*(Nestlé) *Souptime*, French	6 fl. oz.	20
ON*YOS (General Mills)	1 T.	35
ORANGE:		
Peeled	½ cup	62
Sections	4 oz.	35
ORANGE-APRICOT DRINK (Ann Page)	1 cup	125
ORANGE-APRICOT JUICE COCKTAIL, *Musselman's*	8 fl. oz.	100
ORANGE DRINK:		
Canned:		
(Ann Page)	8 fl. oz.	121
(Hi-C)	8 fl. oz.	123
(Lincoln)	8 fl. oz.	128
*Mix (Hi-C)	8 fl. oz.	91
ORANGE EXTRACT:		
(Durkee) imitation	1 tsp.	14
(Virginia Dare)	1 tsp.	22
ORANGE-GRAPEFRUIT JUICE:		
Canned (Del Monte):		
Sweetened	6 fl. oz.	91
Unsweetened	6 fl. oz.	79
*Frozen (Minute Maid) unsweetened	6 fl. oz.	70
ORANGE JUICE:		
Canned:		
(Del Monte) sweetened	6 fl. oz.	76
(Sunkist) unsweetened	½ cup	60
Chilled (Minute Maid)	6 fl. oz.	83
*Frozen:		
Bright & Early, imitation	6 fl. oz.	90
(Minute Maid) unsweetened	6 fl. oz.	86
(Snow Crop)	6 fl. oz.	86
(Sunkist)	6 fl. oz.	92

Food and Description	Measure or Quantity	Calories
ORANGE PEEL, candied	1 oz.	93
ORANGE-PINEAPPLE DRINK, canned:		
(Ann Page)	1 cup	126
(Lincoln)	8 fl. oz.	128
ORANGE-PINEAPPLE JUICE COCKTAIL, *Musselman's*	8 fl. oz.	100
*****ORANGE PLUS** (Birds Eye)	6 fl. oz.	99
ORANGE SPREAD, dietetic (Estee)	1 tsp.	8
OVALTINE, chocolate	¾ oz.	80
OYSTER:		
Raw:		
Eastern	19-31 small or 13-19 med.	158
Pacific & Western	6-9 small or 4-6 med.	218
Canned (Bumble) shelled, whole, solids & liq.	1 cup	218
Fried	4 oz.	271
OYSTER STEW, home recipe	½ cup	103
*****OYSTER STEW SOUP** (Campbell):		
Made with milk	10-oz. serving	170
Made with water	10-oz. serving	70

P

Food and Description	Measure or Quantity	Calories
PANCAKE BATTER, FROZEN:		
*(Aunt Jemima):		
Plain	4″ pancake	70
Blueberry	4″ pancake	68
Buttermilk	4″ pancake	71
*(Rich's):		
Plain	1 pancake	113
Blueberry	⅒ of pkg.	102
Buttermilk	⅒ of pkg.	109
PANCAKE & SAUSAGE, frozen (Swanson)	6-oz. entree	500
*****PANCAKE & WAFFLE MIX:**		
Plain:		
(Aunt Jemima):		
Complete	4″ pancake	67
Original	4″ pancake	73
(Log Cabin):		
Complete	4″ pancake	58
Original	4″ pancake	60
(Pillsbury) *Hungry Jack:*		

Food and Description	Measure or Quantity	Calories
Complete, bulk	4" pancake	63
Complete, packets	4" pancake	60
Extra Lights	4" pancake	67
Panshakes	4" pancake	83
Blueberry (Pillsbury) *Hungry Jack*	4" pancake	110
Buckwheat (Aunt Jemima)	4" pancake	67
Buttermilk:		
(Aunt Jemima):		
Regular	4" pancake	100
Complete	4" pancake	80
(Betty Crocker):		
Regular	4" pancake	93
Complete	4" pancake	70
(Log Cabin)	4" pancake	77
(Pillsbury) *Hungry Jack*, complete	4" pancake	80
Whole wheat (Aunt Jemima)	4" pancake	83
Dietetic (Tillie Lewis) complete	4" pancake	45
PANCAKE & WAFFLE SYRUP (See SYRUP, Pancake & Waffle)		
PAPAYA, fresh:		
Cubed	½ cup	36
Juice	4 oz.	78
PAPRIKA (French's)	1 tsp.	7
PARSLEY:		
Fresh, chopped	1 T.	2
Dried (French's)	1 tsp.	4
PASSION FRUIT, giant, whole	1 lb.	53
PASTINA (Ann Page)	1 oz.	108
PASTOSO (Petri)	3 fl. oz.	71
PASTRAMI:		
(Eckrich) sliced	1-oz. serving	47
(Vienna)	1-oz. serving	86
PASTRY SHELL, frozen (Pepperidge Farm)	1 patty shell	240
PÂTÉ:		
De foie gras	1 T.	69
Liver (Hormel)	1 T.	35
PDQ:		
Chocolate	1 T.	66
Strawberry	1 T.	60
PEA, green:		
Boiled	½ cup	58
Canned, regular pack, solids & liq.:		
(April Showers) early	½ cup	61

Food and Description	Measure or Quantity	Calories
(Del Monte):		
Early	½ cup	52
Seasoned	½ cup	54
(Green Giant):		
Early, with onions	½ cup	61
Sweet	½ cup	52
Sweetlets	½ cup	49
Sweet, with onion	½ cup	52
(Kounty Kist):		
Early	½ cup	71
Sweet	½ cup	64
(Le Sueur) early	½ cup	52
(Libby's) sweet	½ cup	66
(Lindy's) sweet	½ cup	64
(Stokely-Van Camp) early	½ cup	65
Canned, dietetic pack, solids & liq.:		
(Diet Delight)	½ cup	47
(Featherweight) sweet	½ cup	70
(S&W) *Nutradiet*, sweet	½ cup	40
(Tillie Lewis) *Tasti-Diet*	½ cup	40
Frozen:		
(Birds Eye):		
In cream sauce	⅓ of pkg.	134
With sliced mushrooms	⅓ of pkg.	65
Sweet	⅓ of pkg.	70
(Green Giant):		
Creamed, *Bake'n Serve*	⅓ of pkg.	106
Early, small	4-oz. serving	76
Sweet	4½-oz. serving	85
Sweet in butter sauce	⅓ of pkg.	74
(Kounty Kist)	4-oz. serving	100
(McKenzie)	⅓ of pkg.	77
(Seabrook Farms)	⅓ of pkg.	77
(Seabrook Farms) petite	⅓ of pkg.	62
PEA & CARROT:		
Canned, regular pack, solids & liq.:		
(Del Monte)	½ cup	49
(Libby's)	½ cup	56
Canned, dietetic pack, solids & liq.:		
(Diet Delight)	½ cup	36
(S&W) *Nutradiet*	½ cup	35
Frozen (Birds Eye)	⅓ of pkg.	50
PEA & CAULIFLOWER, frozen (Birds Eye)	⅓ of pkg.	67

Food and Description	Measure or Quantity	Calories
PEA & ONION, frozen (Birds Eye)	⅓ pkg.	67
PEA POD:		
Boiled, drained solids	4 oz.	49
Frozen (La Choy)	6-oz. pkg.	90
PEA & POTATO, frozen (Birds Eye) cream sauce	⅓ of pkg.	145
PEA SOUP, GREEN:		
*Canned, regular pack (Campbell)	11-oz. serving	210
Canned, dietetic pack:		
(Campbell) low sodium	7½-oz. can	150
*(Dia-Mel)	8-oz. serving	110
*Mix:		
(Lipton)	1 cup	130
(Nestlé) *Souptime*	6 fl. oz.	70
PEA SOUP, SPLIT, canned:		
*(Ann Page) with ham	1 cup	180
(Campbell):		
Chunky, with ham	19-oz. can	420
*Condensed, with ham & bacon	11-oz. serving	220
PEACH:		
Fresh, with thin skin	2″ peach	38
Fresh, slices	½ cup	32
Canned, regular pack, solids & liq.:		
(Del Monte)		
Cling	½ cup	95
Spiced	½ cup	85
(Libby's):		
Halves, heavy syrup	½ cup	105
Sliced, heavy syrup	½ cup	102
(Stokely-Van Camp)	½ cup	95
Canned, dietetic pack, solids & liq.:		
(Del Monte) *Lite,* Cling	½ cup	53
(Diet Delight):		
Cling, syrup pack	½ cup	60
Cling, water pack	½ cup	30
(Featherweight):		
Cling or Freestone, juice pack	½ cup	50
Cling, water pack	½ cup	30
(Libby's) water pack	½ cup	33
(S&W) *Nutradiet:*		
Cling, juice pack	½ cup	60
Cling, water pack	½ cup	30
Freestone, juice pack	½ cup	50

Food and Description	Measure or Quantity	Calories
(Tillie Lewis) *Tasti-Diet*, Cling	½ cup	54
PEACH BUTTER (Smucker's)	1 T.	45
PEACH DRINK (Hi-C):		
Canned	6 fl. oz.	90
*Mix	6 fl. oz.	72
PEACH ICE CREAM:		
(Breyer's)	¼ pt.	130
(Sealtest) old fashioned	¼ pt.	130
PEACH LIQUEUR (DeKuyper)	1 fl. oz.	82
PEACH PRESERVE OR JAM:		
Sweetened (Smucker's)	1 T.	53
Dietetic:		
(Dia-Mel)	1 T.	6
(Featherweight)	1 T.	16
(Featherweight) artificially sweetened	1 T.	6
(Tillie Lewis) *Tasti-Diet*	1 T.	11
PEANUT:		
Dry roasted:		
(A&P)	1 oz.	176
(Frito-Lay)	1 oz.	173
(Planters)	1 oz.	160
Oil roasted (Planters)	1 oz. (jar)	179
PEANUT BUTTER:		
Regular:		
(Ann Page) krunchy or smooth	1 T.	106
(Jif) creamy	1 T.	93
(Peter Pan):		
Crunchy	1 T.	101
Smooth	1 T.	94
(Planters) crunchy or smooth	1 T.	95
(Skippy):		
Creamy	1 T.	108
Creamy, old fashioned	1 T.	101
Super chunk	1 T.	102
Super chunk, old fashioned	1 T.	101
(Smucker's):		
Creamy or crunchy	1 T.	90
Natural	1 T.	100
(Sultana) regular	1 T.	107
Dietetic:		
(Peter Pan) low sodium	1 T.	106
(S&W) *Nutradiet*, low sodium	1 T.	93
PEANUT BUTTER BAKING CHIPS (Reese's)	3 T. (1 oz.)	151

Food and Description	Measure or Quantity	Calories
PEA PUREE, dietetic (Featherweight)	1 cup	160
PEAR:		
Whole	3" x 2½" pear	101
Canned, regular pack, solids & liq.:		
(Del Monte)	½ cup	88
(Libby's)	½ cup	94
Canned, dietetic pack, solids & liq.:		
(Del Monte) *Lite*	½ cup	58
(Featherweight):		
Bartlett, juice pack	½ cup	60
Bartlett, water pack	½ cup	40
(Libby's) water pack	½ cup	40
(S&W) *Nutradiet:*		
Juice pack	½ cup	60
Water pack	½ cup	35
PEBBLES, cereal:		
Cocoa	⅞ cup	117
Fruity	⅞ cup	116
PECAN:		
Halves	67 peaces	48
Roasted, dry:		
(Flavor House)	1 oz.	195
(Planters)	1 oz.	190
PEP, cereal (Kellogg's)	¾ cup	110
PEPPER:		
Black (French's)	1 tsp.	9
Lemon (Durkee)	1 tsp.	1
Seasoned (French's)	1 tsp.	8
PEPPER, CHILI, canned:		
Old El Paso, green	1-oz. serving	7
(Ortega) hot	1-oz. serving	6
PEPPER, JALAPENO, canned (Ortego)	1-oz. serving	8
PEPPERMINT EXTRACT (Durkee) imitation	1 tsp.	15
PEPPERONI:		
(Hormel) sliced	1-oz. serving	142
(Swift)	1-oz. serving	152
*****PEPPER POT SOUP**, canned (Campbell)	10-oz. serving	120
PEPPER STEAK, frozen:		
*(Chun King) stir fry	⅕ of pkg.	70
(Stouffer's)	5¼-oz. serving	354

Food and Description	Measure or Quantity	Calories
PEPPER, STUFFED:		
Home recipe	2¾″ x 2½″ pepper with 1⅛ cups stuffing	314
Frozen:		
(Green Giant)	7-oz. serving	202
(Weight Watchers) with veal	12-oz. meal	366
PEPPER, SWEET:		
Green, whole	1 med.	13
Red, whole	1 med.	19
PERCH:		
White, meat only	4 oz.	134
Yellow, meat only	4 oz.	103
Frozen:		
(Banquet)	8¾-oz. dinner	434
(Mrs. Paul's) fillets, breaded & fried	2-oz. fillet	127
(Van de Kamp's) batter dipped, french fried	2.3-oz. piece	145
(Weight Watchers)	16-oz. meal	294
PERNOD (Julius Wile)	1 fl. oz.	79
PERSIMMON	4.4-oz. fruit	81
PICKLE:		
Cucumber, fresh or bread & butter:		
(Fanning's)	1 fl. oz.	14
(Featherweight) sliced, no added salt	1 oz.	12
(Nalley's) chips	1 oz.	27
Dill:		
(Featherweight) whole, low sodium	1 oz.	4
(Nalley's) regular & Polish style	1 oz.	3
(Smucker's):		
Candied sticks	4″ stick	45
Hamburger sliced	1 slice	<1
Polish, whole	3½″ pickle	8
Spears	3½″ spear	6
Hamburger (Nalley's) chips	1 oz.	3
Kosher dill:		
(Claussen) halves or whole	2 oz.	7
(Featherweight) low sodium	1 oz.	4
(Nalley's)	2 oz.	12
(Smucker's):		
Baby	2¾″ pickle	4

Food and Description	Measure or Quantity	Calories
Slices	1 slice	<1
Whole	2½" pickle	8
Sweet:		
(Nalley's):		
Regular	1 oz.	37
Nubbins	1 oz.	28
(Smucker's):		
Candied mix	1 piece	14
Gherkins	2" pickle	15
Whole	2½" pickle	18
Sweet & sour (Claussen) slices	1 slice	3
PIE:		
Regular:		
Apple:		
Home recipe, two-crust	⅙ of 9" pie	404
(Hostess)	4½-oz. pie	409
(Tastykake)	4-oz. pie	348
(Tastykake) French	4¼-oz. pie	405
Banana, home recipe, cream or custard	⅙ of 9" pie	336
Berry (Hostess)	4½-oz. pie	404
Blackberry, home recipe, two-crust	⅙ of 9" pie	384
Blueberry:		
Home recipe, two-crust	⅙ of 9" pie	382
(Hostess)	4½-oz. pie	394
(Tastykake)	4-oz. pie	366
Boston cream, home recipe	1/12 of 8" pie	208
Butterscotch, home recipe, one-crust	⅙ of 9" pie	406
Cherry:		
Home recipe, two-crust	⅙ of 9" pie	412
(Hostess)	4½-oz. pie	435
(Tastykake)	4-oz. pie	381
Chocolate chiffon, home recipe	⅙ of 9" pie	459
Chocolate meringue, home recipe	⅙ of 9" pie	353
Coconut custard, home recipe	⅙ of 9" pie	357
Lemon (Hostess)	4½-oz. pie	415
Mince, home recipe, two-crust	⅙ of 9" pie	428
Peach:		
(Hostess)	4½-oz. pie	409
(Tastykake)	4-oz. pie	349
Pecan (Frito-Lay)	3-oz. serving	353
Pumpkin, home recipe, one-crust	⅙ of 9" pie	321

Food and Description	Measure or Quantity	Calories
Raisin, home recipe, two-crust	⅙ of 9" pie	427
Rhubarb, home recipe, two-crust	⅙ of 9" pie	400
Frozen:		
Apple:		
(Banquet)	⅙ of 20-oz. pie	288
(Morton):		
Regular	⅙ of 24-oz. pie	295
Great Little Desserts	8-oz. pie	598
Great Little Desserts, Dutch	7.8-oz. pie	607
(Sara Lee):		
Regular	⅙ of 31-oz. pie	376
Dutch	⅙ of 30-oz. pie	354
Banana cream:		
(Banquet)	⅙ of 14-oz. pie	172
(Morton):		
Regular	⅙ of 16-oz. pie	174
Great Little Desserts	3½-oz. pie	237
Blueberry:		
(Banquet)	⅙ of 20-oz. pie	253
(Morton):		
Regular	⅙ of 24-oz. pie	286
Great Little Desserts	8-oz. pie	589
(Sara Lee)	⅙ of 31-oz. pie	449
Cherry:		
(Banquet)	⅙ of 20-oz. pie	228
(Morton):		
Regular	⅙ of 24-oz. pie	300
Great Little Desserts	8-oz. pie	589
(Sara Lee)	⅙ of 31-oz. pie	397
Chocolate cream:		
(Banquet)	⅙ of 14-oz. pie	177
(Morton):		
Regular	⅙ of 16-oz. pie	199
Great Little Desserts	2½-oz. pie	266
Coconut cream:		
(Banquet)	⅙ of 14-oz. pie	178
(Morton):		
Regular	⅙ of 16-oz. pie	197
Great Little Desserts	2½-oz. pie	266
Coconut custard:		
(Banquet)	⅙ of 20-oz. pie	203
(Morton) *Great Little Desserts*	6½-oz. pie	369

Food and Description	Measure or Quantity	Calories
Custard (Banquet)	1/8 of 20-oz. pie	247
Lemon cream:		
(Banquet)	1/8 of 14-oz. pie	168
(Morton):		
Regular	1/8 of 16-oz. pie	182
Great Little Desserts	3½-oz. pie	245
Mince:		
(Banquet)	1/8 of 20-oz. pie	252
(Morton)	1/8 of 24-oz. pie	314
Neapolitan (Morton)	1/8 of 16-oz. pie	195
Peach:		
(Banquet)	1/8 of 20-oz. pie	263
(Morton)	1/8 of 24-oz. pie	286
(Sara Lee)	1/8 of 31 oz. pie	458
Pumpkin:		
(Banquet)	1/8 of 20-oz. pie	206
(Morton)	1/8 of 24-oz. pie	235
(Sara Lee)	1/8 of 45-oz. pie	354
Strawberry cream:		
(Banquet)	1/8 of 14-oz. pie	169
(Morton)	1/8 of 16-oz. pie	182
PIECRUST, home recipe, 9″ pie	1 crust	900
*PIECRUST MIX:		
(Betty Crocker) regular or stick:		
Regular	1/16 pkg.	120
Stick	1/8 stick	120
(Flako)	1/6 of 9″ pie shell	260
(Pillsbury) mix or stick	1/6 of 2-crust shell	290
PIE FILLING (See also PUDDING OR PIE FILLING):		
Apple (Comstock)	1/6 of 21-oz. can	110
Apple rings or slices (See APPLE, canned)		
Apricot (Comstock)	1/6 of 21-oz. can	110
Banana cream (Comstock)	1/6 of 21-oz. can	110
Blueberry (Comstock)	1/6 of 21-oz. can	120
Cherry (Comstock)	1/6 of 21-oz. can	120
Chocolate (Comstock)	1/6 of 21-oz. can	140
Coconut cream (Comstock)	1/6 of 21-oz. can	120
Coconut custard, home recipe, made with egg yolk & milk	5 oz. (inc. crust)	288
Lemon (Comstock)	1/6 of 21-oz. can	160
Mincemeat (Comstock)	1/6 of 21-oz. can	170
Peach (Comstock)	1/6 of 21-oz. can	130

Food and Description	Measure or Quantity	Calories
Pineapple (Comstock)	⅙ of 21-oz. can	110
Pumpkin (Comstock) (See also PUMPKIN, canned)	⅙ of 27-oz. can	170
Raisin (Comstock)	⅙ of 21-oz. can	140
Strawberry (Comstock)	⅙ of 21-oz. can	130
*PIE MIX (Betty Crocker) Boston cream	⅛ of pie	260
PIGS FEET, pickled	4 oz.	226
PIMIENTO, canned:		
(Dromedary)	1-oz. serving	10
(Ortega)	¼ cup	6
PIÑA COLADA:		
Canned:		
(Mr. Boston) 12½% alcohol	3 fl. oz.	240
(Party Tyme) 12½% alcohol	3 fl. oz.	94
Mix:		
Dry (Party Tyme)	½-oz. pkg.	50
Liquid (Holland House)	2 fl. oz.	120
PINEAPPLE:		
Fresh, chunks	½ cup	52
Canned, regular pack, solids & liq.:		
(Del Monte) slices, medium	½ cup	92
(Dole):		
Chunk, crushed, or sliced, juice pack	½ cup	70
Chunk, crushed, or sliced, heavy syrup	½ cup	94
Canned, unsweetened or dietetic, solids & liq.:		
(Del Monte):		
Chunks, juice pack	½ cup	70
Crushed, juice pack	½ cup	77
Slices, juice pack	½ cup	81
(Diet Delight)	½ cup	79
(Featherweight):		
Juice pack	½ cup	70
Water pack	½ cup	60
(S&W) *Nutradiet*, slices	1 slice	30
(Tillie Lewis) *Tasti-Diet*:		
Juice pack	½ cup	72
Water pack	½ cup	60
PINEAPPLE, CANDIED	1 oz.	90
PINEAPPLE FLAVORING (Durkee) imitation	1 tsp.	6

Food and Description	Measure or Quantity	Calories
PINEAPPLE & GRAPEFRUIT JUICE DRINK, canned:		
(Del Monte) regular or pink	6 fl. oz.	98
(Dole) pink	6 fl. oz.	101
PINEAPPLE JUICE:		
Canned:		
(Del Monte) with vitamin C	6 fl. oz.	108
(Dole)	6 fl. oz.	103
*Frozen (Minute Maid)	6 fl. oz.	92
PINEAPPLE-ORANGE DRINK, canned (Hi-C)	6 fl. oz.	94
PINEAPPLE-ORANGE JUICE:		
Canned (Del Monte)	6 fl. oz.	97
*Frozen (Minute Maid)	6 fl. oz.	94
PINEAPPLE PRESERVE or JAM, sweetened (Smucker's)	1 T.	53
PINE NUT, pignolias, shelled	1 oz.	156
PISTACHIO NUT:		
In shell	½ cup	197
Shelled	¼ cup	184
PIZZA PIE:		
Regular, non-frozen:		
Home recipe	⅛ of 14" pie	177
(Pizza Hut):		
Cheese	½ of 10" pie	436
Pepperoni	½ of 10" pie	459
Pork	½ of 10" pie	475
Frozen:		
Cheese:		
(Celeste)	½ of 7-oz. pie	245
(Celeste)	¼ of 19-oz. pie	320
(La Pizzeria):		
Regular	¼ of 20-oz. pie	290
Thick crust	⅓ of 18½-oz. pie	410
(Stouffer's) French bread	½ of 10½-oz. pkg.	327
Tostino's	½ of pie	440
(Weight Watchers)	6-oz. pie	386
Combination:		
(La Pizzeria)	½ of 13½-oz. pie	420
(La Pizzeria)	¼ of 24½-oz. pie	380
Tostino's, classic	⅓ of pie	520
(Van de Kamp's) thick crust	¼ of 23.4-oz. pie	310
Deluxe:		
(Celeste)	½ of 9-oz. pie	298
(Celeste)	¼ of 23½-oz. pie	367
(Stouffer's) French bread	½ of 12⅜-oz. pkg.	404

Food and Description	*Measure or Quantity*	*Calories*
Hamburger (Stouffer's) French bread	½ of 12¼-oz. pkg.	397
Pepperoni:		
(Celeste)	½ of 7¼-oz. pie	264
(Celeste)	¼ of 20-oz. pie	356
(La Pizzeria)	¼ of 21-oz. pie	330
(Stouffer's) French bread	½ of 11¼-oz. pkg.	401
Tostino's	½ of pie	460
(Van de Kamp's) thick crust	¼ of 22-oz. pie	370
Sausage:		
(Celeste)	½ of 8-oz. pie	281
(Celeste)	¼ of 22-oz. pie	375
(La Pizzeria)	½ of 13-oz. pie	430
(Stouffer's) French bread	½ of 12-oz. pkg.	417
Tostino's	½ of pie	470
Tostino's, deep crust	⅙ of pie	300
(Weight Watchers)	6-oz. pie	330
Sausage & mushroom:		
(Celeste)	½ of 9-oz. pie	285
(Celeste)	¼ of 24-oz. pie	379
(Stouffer's) French bread	½ of 12½-oz. pkg.	388
Sicilian style (Celeste):		
Cheese	¼ of 20-oz. pie	329
Deluxe	¼ of 26-oz. pie	425
Sausage	¼ of 24-oz. pie	399
PIZZA PIE MIX:		
Regular (Jeno's)	½ of pkg.	420
Cheese:		
(Jeno's)	½ of pkg.	420
Skillet Pizza (General Mills)	¼ pkg.	210
Pepperoni:		
(Jeno's)	½ of pkg.	510
Skillet Pizza (General Mills)	¼ of pkg.	220
Sausage, *Skillet Pizza* (General Mills)	¼ of pkg.	230
PIZZA ROLL (Jeno's) 12 to pkg.:		
Cheeseburger	½-oz. roll	45
Sausage	½-oz. roll	43
Shrimp & cheese	½-oz. roll	37
PIZZA SAUCE:		
(Contadina)	8-oz. serving	130
(Ragu)	5-oz. serving	120
PIZZA SEASONING SPICE (French's)	1 tsp.	4

Food and Description	Measure or Quantity	Calories
PLUM:		
Fresh, Japanese & hybrid	2" plum	27
Fresh, prune-type, halves	½ cup	60
Canned, regular pack (Stokely-Van Camp)	½ cup	120
Canned, purple, unsweetened or dietetic, solids & liq.:		
(Diet Delight)	½ cup	77
(Featherweight)		
Juice pack	½ cup	80
Water pack	½ cup	40
(S&W) *Nutradiet*, juice pack	½ cup	80
(Tillie Lewis) *Tasti-Diet*	½ cup	73
PLUM PRESERVE OR JAM, sweetened (Smucker's)	1 T.	53
P. M. FRUIT DRINK (Mott's)	6 fl. oz.	90
POLISH-STYLE SAUSAGE (Vienna)	3-oz. piece	240
POLYNESIAN-STYLE DINNER, frozen (Swanson) TV Brand	13-oz. dinner	490
POMEGRANATE, whole	1 lb.	160
POPCORN:		
*Plain:		
(Jiffy Pop)	½ of 5-oz. pkg.	244
(Pillsbury) Microwave Popcorn	1 cup	60
Buttered (Old London)	1 cup	57
Caramel-coated (Bachman)	1-oz. serving	130
(Old London):		
Without peanuts	1¾-oz. bag	195
With peanuts	1 cup	142
With cheese	¾-oz. bag	90
Cheese flavored (Bachman)	1-oz. serving	180
Cracker Jack	¾-oz. serving	90
POPOVER MIX (Flako)	1 popover	170
POPPY SEED (French's)	1 tsp.	13
POPSICLE, twin pop	3-fl.-oz. pop	70
POP TARTS (See TOASTER CAKE or PASTRY)		
PORK:		
Fresh:		
Chop:		
Broiled, lean & fat	3-oz. chop (weighed without bone)	332
Broiled, lean only	3-oz. chop (weighed without bone)	230

Food and Description	Measure or Quantity	Calories
Loin:		
Roasted, lean & fat	3 oz.	308
Roasted, lean only	3 oz.	216
Spareribs, braised	3 oz.	374
Cured ham:		
Roasted, lean & fat	3 oz.	246
Roasted, lean only	3 oz.	159
PORK DINNER (Swanson)		
TV Brand	11¼-oz. dinner	470
PORK RINDS, *Baken-Ets*	1-oz. serving	150
PORK SAUSAGE, cooked		
(Oscar Mayer) *Little Friers*	1 link	61
PORK STEAK, BREADED,		
frozen (Hormel)	3-oz. serving	223
PORK, SWEET & SOUR, frozen:		
(Chun King)	½ of 15-oz. pkg.	220
(La Choy)	½ of 15-oz. pkg.	229
PORT WINE:		
(Gallo)	3 fl. oz.	94
(Great Western)	3 fl. oz.	138
(Louis M. Martini)	6 fl. oz.	165
*****POSTUM**, instant	6 fl. oz.	8
POTATO:		
Cooked:		
Au gratin	½ cup	127
Baked, peeled	2½" dia. potato	92
Boiled, peeled	4.2-oz. potato	79
French-fried	10 pieces	156
Hash-browned, home recipe	½ cup	223
Mashed, milk & butter added	½ cup	92
Canned (Del Monte) drained	1 cup	265
Frozen:		
(Bird's Eye):		
Crinkle cuts	3-oz. serving	115
French fries	3-oz. serving	113
Hash browns	¼ of 16-oz. pkg.	70
Tasti Puffs	¼ of 10-oz. pkg.	190
Tiny Taters	⅙ of 16-oz. pkg.	200
(Green Giant)		
Au gratin, *Bake 'n Serve*	⅓ of 10-oz. pkg.	141
Diced, in sour cream sauce	1 cup	270
Stuffed with cheese-flavored topping	5-oz. entree	240
(Ore-Ida):		
Cottage fries	3.2-oz. serving	149
Crispers	3.2-oz. serving	245
Golden Crinkles	3.2-oz. serving	138

Food and Description	Measure or Quantity	Calories
Golden Fries	3.2-oz. serving	138
Hash browns, shredded	6-oz. serving	120
Hash browns, Southern style, with butter sauce	3-oz. serving	120
O'Brien potatoes	3-oz. serving	60
Shoestrings	3.3-oz. serving	187
Whole, small, peeled	3.2-oz. serving	74
(McKenzie) whole, boiled	3½-oz. serving	69
(Seabrook Farms) whole, boiled	3½-oz. serving	69
(Stouffer's)		
Au gratin	⅓ of pkg.	135
Scalloped	⅓ of pkg.	130
POTATO & BACON, canned (Hormel) *Short Orders*, au gratin	7½-oz. can	230
POTATO & BEEF, canned, *Dinty Moore*, *Short Orders*, hashed	1½-oz. can	250
POTATO CHIP:		
(Bachman)	1 oz.	140
(Frito-Lay's)	1 oz.	157
Lay's	1 oz.	150
Lay's, sour cream & onion flavor	1 oz.	160
(Planter's) stackabel	1 oz.	150
Pringle's	1 oz.	150
POTATO & HAM, canned (Hormel) *Short Orders*, scalloped	7½-oz. can	250
*POTATO MIX:		
Au gratin:		
(Betty Crocker)	½ cup	150
(French's) *Big Tate*	½ cup	160
Creamed (Betty Crocker)	½ cup	160
Hash browns:		
(Betty Crocker) with onion	½ cup	150
(French's) *Big Tate*	½ cup	165
Julienne (Betty Crocker) with milk cheese sauce	½ cup	140
Mashed:		
(American Beauty)	½ cup	140
(Betty Crocker) *Buds*	½ cup	130
(French's) *Big Tate*	½ cup	140
(Pillsbury) *Hungry Jack*, flakes	½ cup	140
Scalloped:		
(Betty Crocker)	½ cup	90
(French's) *Big Tate*	½ cup	160

Food and Description	Measure or Quantity	Calories
Sour cream & chive (Betty Crocker)	½ cup	140
*POTATO PANCAKE MIX (French's) *Big Tate*	3" pancake	43
POTATO SALAD:		
Home recipe	½ cup	181
Canned (Nalley's):		
Regular	4-oz. serving	139
German style	4-oz. serving	143
*POTATO SOUP (Campbell)	10-oz. serving	90
POTATO STICK (Durkee) *O & C*	1½-oz. can	231
POUND CAKE (See CAKE, Pound)		
PRESERVE OR JAM:		
(Ann Page) all flavors	1 T.	57
(Crosse & Blackwell)	1 T.	60
PRETZEL:		
(Bachman):		
Nutzel	1 oz.	110
Thins	1 oz.	110
(Nabisco) *Mister Salty*, Dutch	1 piece	55
(Pepperidge Farm):		
Nuggets	1¼-oz. serving	148
Sticks, thin	1¼-oz. serving	145
Twists, tiny	1 oz.	116
Rold Gold, twists	1 oz.	100
PRODUCT 19, cereal (Kellogg's)	¾ cup	110
PRUNE:		
Dried, cooked	8 prunes & 5 T. liq.	252
Canned, regular (Sunsweet)	5–6 prunes	138
Canned, dietetic (Featherweight) stewed, water pack	½ cup	130
PRUNE JUICE:		
(Del Monte)	6 fl. oz.	137
(Mott's)	6 fl. oz.	140
(Mott's) with prune pulp	6 fl. oz.	120
PRUNE NECTAR, canned (Mott's)	6 fl. oz.	100
PRUNE WHIP, home recipe	½ cup	106
PUDDING OR PIE FILLING:		
Canned, regular pack:		
Banana:		
(Del Monte)	5-oz. container	183
(Hunt's) *Snack Pack*	5-oz. container	180
Butterscotch:		
(Del Monte)	5-oz. container	185
(Hunt's) *Snack Pack*	5-oz. container	170

Food and Description	*Measure or Quantity*	*Calories*
Chocolate:		
(Betty Crocker)	5-oz. container	180
(Del Monte)	5-oz. container	173
(Hunt's) *Snack Pack*	5-oz. container	180
Lemon (Hunt's) *Snack Pack*	5-oz. container	150
Rice:		
(Betty Crocker)	½ cup	150
(Comstock)	½ of 7½-oz. can	120
(Hunt's) *Snack Pack*	5-oz. container	190
(Menner's)	½ of 7½-oz. can	120
Tapioca:		
(Betty Crocker)	½ cup	150
(Del Monte)	5-oz. container	174
(Hunt's) *Snack Pack*	5-oz. container	140
Vanilla:		
(Del Monte)	5-oz. container	189
(Hunt's) *Snack Pack*	5-oz. container	180
Canned, dietetic pack (Sego) all flavors	4-oz. serving	125
Chilled, *Swiss Miss:*		
Butterscotch	4½-oz. container	174
Chocolate	4½-oz. container	180
Tapioca	4½-oz. container	176
Vanilla	4½-oz. container	192
Frozen (Rich's):		
Banana	3-oz. container	142
Butterscotch	4½-oz. container	199
Chocolate	4½-oz. container	214
Vanilla	4½-oz. container	199
Mix, sweetened, regular & instant:		
Banana:		
(Ann Page) regular	¼ of 3⅛-oz. pkg.	84
*(Jell-O) regular	⅙ of 9" pie, excluding crust	110
*(Jell-O) cream, instant	½ cup	180
*(Royal) regular	½ cup	160
*(Royal) instant	½ cup	180
*Butter Pecan (Jell-O) instant	½ cup	180
Butterscotch:		
(Ann Page) regular	¼ of 3⅝-oz. pkg.	96
*(Jell-O) regular or instant	½ cup	180
*(My-T-Fine) regular	½ cup	143
*(Royal) regular	½ cup	160
*(Royal) instant	½ cup	180
Chocolate:		
*(Jell-O) regular	½ cup	180

Food and Description	Measure or Quantity	Calories
*(Jell-O) instant	½ cup	190
*(My-T-Fine) regular	½ cup	169
*(My-T-Fine) fudge, regular	½ cup	151
*(Royal) regular	½ cup	180
*(Royal) instant	½ cup	190
Coconut:		
(Ann Page)	¼ of 3½-oz. pkg.	100
*(Jell-O) cream, regular	⅙ of 9" pie, excluding crust	110
*(Royal) instant	½ cup	170
*Coffee (Royal) instant	½ cup	180
Custard:		
(Ann Page) egg, regular	¼ of 2¾-oz. pkg.	73
*Jell-O Americana, egg, golden	½ cup	170
*(Royal) regular	½ cup	150
*Flan (Royal) regular	½ cup	150
Lemon:		
(Ann Page) regular	¼ of 3-oz. pkg.	80
*(Jell-O) instant	½ cup	180
*(My-T-Fine) regular	½ cup	164
*(Royal) regular	½ cup	160
*(Royal) instant	½ cup	180
*Lime (Royal) Key Lime, regular	½ cup	160
*Pineapple (Jell-O) cream, instant	½ cup	180
Pistachio:		
*(Jell-O) instant	½ cup	190
*(Royal) nut, instant	½ cup	170
*Rice, *Jell-O Americana*	½ cup	180
Tapioca:		
*Jell-O Americana, chocolate or vanilla	½ cup	160
*(My-T-Fine) vanilla	½ cup	130
*(Royal) vanilla	½ cup	160
Vanilla:		
*(Jell-O) regular	½ cup	160
*(Jell-O) French, regular & instant	½ cup	180
*(My-T-Fine) regular	½ cup	133
*(Royal) regular	½ cup	160
*(Royal) instant	½ cup	180
*Mix, dietetic:		
Butterscotch:		
(D-Zerta)	½ cup	70

Food and Description	Measure or Quantity	Calories
(Featherweight) artificially sweetened	½ cup	50
Chocolate:		
(Dia-Mel)	4-oz. serving	60
(D-Zerta)	½ cup	70
(Estee)	½ cup	48
(Featherweight) artificially sweetened	½ cup	60
Lemon:		
(Dia-Mel)	½ cup	53
(Estee)	½ cup	106
Vanilla:		
(D-Zerta)	½ cup	70
(Estee)	½ cup	39
(Featherweight) artificially sweetened	½ cup	50
PUFFED RICE:		
(Malt-O-Meal)	1 cup	52
(Quaker)	1 cup	55
PUFFED WHEAT:		
(Malt-O-Meal)	1 cup	48
(Quaker)	1 cup	54
PUFFS, frozen (Rich's) vanilla	1 puff	167
PUMPKIN SEED, in hull	1 oz.	116

Q

QUAIL, raw, meat & skin	4 oz.	195
QUIK (Nestlé) chocolate or strawberry	1 tsp.	45
QUISP, cereal	1⅛ cups	121

R

RADISH	2 small radishes	4
RAISIN, dried:		
(Del Monte)	3 oz.	287
(Sun-Maid)	3 oz.	250
RAISINS, RICE & RYE, cereal (Kellogg's)	1 cup	140
RALSTON, cereal	¼ cup	90
RASPBERRY:		
Fresh:		
Black, trimmed	½ cup	49
Red, trimmed	½ cup	41
Frozen (Birds Eye) quick thaw	5-oz. serving	145

Food and Description	Measure or Quantity	Calories
RASPBERRY PRESERVE or JAM:		
Sweetened (Smucker's)	1 T.	53
Dietetic:		
(Dia-Mel) black	1 T.	6
(Featherweight) red	1 T.	16
(S&W) *Nutradiet*, red	1 T.	12
RASPBERRY SPREAD, low sugar (Smucker's)	1 T.	24
RAVIOLI:		
Canned, regular pack:		
(Franco-American):		
Beef, *Raviolios*	7½-oz. serving	209
Cheese, in tomato sauce	7½-oz. can	260
(Nalley's) beef	8-oz. serving	214
Canned, dietetic (Dia-Mel) beef, in sauce	8-oz. c.	230
RELISH:		
Hamburger (Nalley's)	1 T.	17
Hot dog (Nalley's)	1 T.	24
Sweet (Smucker's)	1 T.	23
Dietetic (Featherweight) sweet	1 oz.	11
RHINE WINE:		
(Great Western)	3 fl. oz.	73
(Inglenook) Navalle	3 fl. oz.	76
(Taylor)	3 fl. oz.	75
RHUBARB, cooked, sweetened	½ cup	169
RICE:		
*Brown (Uncle Ben's) parboiled, with added butter	⅔ cup	152
*White:		
(Minute Rice) instant, no added butter	⅔ cup	120
(Success) long grain	½ cooking bag	110
*White & wild (Carolina)	½ cup	90
RICE CHEX, cereal	1⅛ cups	110
RICE, FRIED:		
*Canned (La Choy):		
Chicken	½ cup	209
Chinese style	½ cup	207
Frozen:		
(La Choy) & pork	6-oz. serving	245
(Temple) & shrimp	1 cup	297
RICE, FRIED, SEASONING MIX (Durkee)	1 cup	213
RICE KRISPIES, cereal (Kellogg's)	1 cup	110

Food and Description	*Measure or Quantity*	*Calories*
RICE MIX:		
Beef:		
*(Carolina) *Bake-It-Easy*	¼ of pkg.	110
Rice-A-Roni	⅙ of 8-oz. pkg.	129
Chicken:		
*(Carolina) *Bake-It-Easy*	¼ of pkg.	110
Rice-A-Roni	⅙ of 8-oz. pkg.	160
*Drumstick (Minute Rice)	½ cup	150
*Fried (Minute Rice)	½ cup	160
*Long grain & wild (Uncle Ben's) with added butter	½ cup	112
*Oriental (Carolina) *Bake-It-Easy*	½ of pkg.	120
*Rib roast (Minute Rice)	½ cup	150
Spanish:		
*(Carolina) *Bake-It-Easy*	¼ of pkg.	110
*(Minute Rice)	½ cup	150
Rice-A-Roni	⅙ of 7½-oz. pkg.	124
RICE, SPANISH, canned:		
(Comstock)	½ of 7½-oz. can	140
(Libby's)	7½-oz. serving	135
(Menner's)	½ of 7½-oz. can	140
(Van Camp)	½ cup	95
RICE & VEGETABLE, frozen:		
(Birds Eye) with peas & mushrooms	⅓ of pkg.	106
(Green Giant):		
& broccoli in cheese sauce	½ of 11-oz. pkg.	140
Continental, with green bean & almonds	½ of 11-oz. pkg.	138
Medley, with peas & mushrooms	½ of 11-oz. pkg.	141
Pilaf, with mushrooms & onions	½ of 11-oz. pkg.	141
Verdi, with bell pepper & parsley	½ of 11-oz. pkg.	175
RICE WINE:		
Chinese, 20.7% alcohol	1 fl. oz.	38
Japanese, 10.6% alcohol	1 fl. oz.	72
Non-alcoholic	1 fl. oz.	30
RIESLING WINE, Grey (Inglenook)	3 fl. oz.	60
ROCK & RYE (Mr. Boston)	1 fl. oz.	7
ROE, baked or broiled, cod & shad	4 oz.	143
ROLL OR BUN:		
Commercial type, non-frozen:		
Biscuit (Wonder)	1 roll	214
Brown & serve (Wonder) *Gem Style*	1 roll	86
Commercial type, non-frozen:		
Club (Pepperidge Farm)	1 roll	100

Food and Description	Measure or Quantity	Calories
Crescent (Pepperidge Farm) butter	1 roll	120
Deli-twist (Arnold)	1 roll	110
Dinner:		
Home Pride	1-oz. roll	93
(Pepperidge Farm)	1 roll	60
(Wonder)	2½-oz. roll	214
Finger:		
(Arnold) *Dinner Party*	1 roll	55
(Pepperidge Farm) sesame	1 roll	57
(Pepperidge Farm) white	1 roll	53
Frankfurter:		
(Arnold) Hot Dog	1 roll	110
(Wonder)	2-oz. roll	162
French:		
(Arnold) *Francisco,* Sourdough	1 roll	90
(Pepperidge Farm):		
Small	1 roll	240
Large	1 roll	380
Golden Twist (Pepperidge Farm)	1 roll	110
Hamburger:		
(Arnold)	1 roll	110
(Pepperidge Farm)	1 roll	120
Hearth (Pepperidge Farm)	1 roll	55
Honey (Hostess)	1 cake	579
Kaiser-Hogie (Wonder)	1 roll	465
Old fashioned (Pepperidge Farm)	1 roll	53
Parkerhouse:		
(Arnold) *Dinner Party*	1 roll	55
(Pepperidge Farm)	1 roll	57
Party pan (Pepperidge Farm)	1 roll	33
Sandwich (Arnold) soft	1 roll	110
Sesame crisp (Pepperidge Farm)	1 roll	63
Frozen:		
Apple crunch (Sara Lee)	1-oz. roll	102
Caramel pecan (Sara Lee)	1.3-oz. roll	161
Caramel sticky (Sara Lee)	1-oz. bun	116
Cinnamon (Sara Lee)	.9-oz. roll	100
Croissant (Sara Lee)	.9-oz. roll	109
Crumb (Sara Lee):		
Blueberry	1¾-oz. piece	169
French	1¾-oz. piece	188

Food and Description	Measure or Quantity	Calories
Danish (Sara Lee):		
Apple	1.3-oz. roll	120
Apple Country	1.8-oz. roll	156
Cheese	1.3-oz. roll	130
Cheese Country	1½-oz. roll	146
Cherry	1.3-oz. roll	125
Cherry Country	1.6-oz. roll	135
Cinnamon Raisin	1.3-oz. roll	147
Pecan	1.3-oz. roll	148
Honey:		
(Morton):		
Regular	2½-oz. roll	231
Mini	1.3-oz. roll	133
(Sara Lee)	1-oz. roll	109
ROLL or BUN DOUGH:		
*Frozen (Rich's) onion	2½-oz. roll	196
Caramel danish, with nuts	1 roll	150
Cinnamon with icing, *Ballard*	1 roll	100
Cinnamon raisin danish	1 roll	135
Crescent	1 roll	200
Wheat, Bakery Style	1 roll	90
White, Bakery Style	1 roll	90
*ROLL MIX, HOT (Pillsbury)	1 roll	95
ROSEMARY LEAVES (French's)	1 tsp.	5
ROSÉ WINE:		
(Great Western)	3 fl. oz.	80
(Inglenook) Gamay or Vintage	3 fl. oz.	60
ROTINI IN TOMATO SAUCE, canned (Franco-American):		
Plain	7½-oz. can	200
With meatball	7⅜-oz. can	240
RUM EXTRACT (Durkee) imitation	1 tsp.	14
RUTABAGA, boiled, diced	½ cup	30

S

SAFFLOWER SEED, in hull	1 oz.	89
SAGE (French's)	1 tsp.	4
SAKE WINE	1 fl. oz.	39
SALAD DRESSING:		
Regular:		
Avocado Goddess (Marie's)	1 T.	95
Bacon (Seven Seas) creamy	1 T.	60
Bell pepper (Seven Seas) *Viva*	1 T.	45

Food and Description	Measure or Quantity	Calories
Bleu or blue cheese:		
(Bernstein) Danish	1 T.	60
(Seven Seas) chunky	1 T.	70
(Wish-Bone) chunky	1 T.	80
Caesar:		
(Pfeiffer)	1 T.	70
(Seven Seas) *Viva*	1 T.	60
(Wish-Bone)	1 T.	80
Capri (Seven Seas)	1 T.	70
French:		
(Bernstein's) creamy	1 T.	56
(Pfeiffer)	1 T.	55
(Seven Seas) creamy	1 T.	60
(Wish-Bone) deluxe	1 T.	50
Garlic (Wish-Bone) creamy	1 T.	80
Green Goddess:		
(Seven Seas)	1 T.	60
(Wish-Bone)	1 T.	70
Herb & spice (Seven Seas)	1 T.	60
Italian:		
(Bernstein's)	1 T.	50
(Marie's)	1 T.	100
(Pfeiffer) chef	1 T.	60
(Seven Seas)	1 T.	70
(Wish-Bone)	1 T.	80
Louis Dressing (Nalley's)	1 T.	69
Onion (Wish-Bone) California	1 T.	80
Onion 'N Chive (Seven Seas) creamy	1 T.	60
Red wine vinegar & oil (Seven Seas)	1 T.	60
Roquefort:		
(Bernstein's)	1 T.	65
(Marie's)	1 T.	105
Russian:		
(Pfeiffer)	1 T.	65
(Seven Seas) creamy	1 T.	80
Sesame (Sahadi):		
Creamy	1 T.	60
Spice	1 T.	80
Spin Blend (Hellmann's)	1 T.	56
Sweet'N Sour (Dutch Pantry) creamy	1 T.	77
Thousand Island:		
(Pfeiffer)	1 T.	65
(Seven Seas)	1 T.	50
Vinaigrette (Bernstein's) French	1 T.	49

Food and Description	Measure or Quantity	Calories
Dietetic:		
Bleu or blue cheese:		
(Dia-Mel)	1 T.	15
(Featherweight) imitation	1 T.	4
(Tillie Lewis) *Tasti-Diet*	1 T.	11
Caesar:		
(Dia-Mel)	1 T.	50
(Estee) garlic	1 T.	4
(Pfeiffer)	1 T.	10
Cucumber & onion (Featherweight) creamy	1 T.	4
French:		
(Pfeiffer)	1 T.	16
(Wish-Bone)	1 T.	25
Italian:		
(Dia-Mel)	1 T.	2
(Estee) spicy	1 T.	4
(Featherweight)	1 T.	4
(Pfeiffer)	1 T.	10
(Weight Watchers)	1 T.	50
(Wish-Bone)	1 T.	20
Red wine (Pfeiffer)	1 T.	10
Russian:		
(Dia-Mel)	1 T.	9
(Featherweight) creamy	1 T.	6
(Pfeiffer)	1 T.	15
(Tillie Lewis) *Tasti-Diet*	1 T.	12
(Weight Watchers)	1 T.	50
(Wish-Bone)	1 T.	25
Thousand Island:		
(Dia-Mel)	1 T.	30
(Pfeiffer)	1 T.	15
(Weight Watchers)	1 T.	50
(Wish-Bone)	1 T.	25
2-Calorie Low Sodium (Featherweight)	1 T.	2
Whipped:		
(Dia-Mel)	1 T.	22
(Tillie Lewis) *Tasti-Diet*	1 T.	23
SALAD DRESSING MIX:		
*Regular (Good Seasons):		
Bleu or blue cheese:		
Regular	1 T.	90
Thick'n Creamy	1 T.	80
Buttermilk Farm Style	1 T.	60
French:		
Old fashioned	1 T.	80

Food and Description	Measure or Quantity	Calories
Thick'n Creamy	1 T.	75
Garlic	1 T.	80
Italian	1 T.	80
Onion	1 T.	80
Thousand Island, *Thick'n Creamy*	1 T.	75
Dietetic:		
*Blue cheese (Weight Watchers)	1 T.	10
French:		
(Dia-Mel)	½-oz. pkg.	18
*(Weight Watchers)	1 T.	4
Garlic (Dia-Mel)	½-oz. pkg.	21
Italian:		
(Dia-Mel)	½-oz. pkg.	2
*(Good Seasons)	1 T.	8
*(Weight Watchers):		
Regular	1 T.	2
Creamy	1 T.	4
Russian:		
(Louis Sherry)	½-oz. packet	20
*(Weight Watchers)	1 T.	4
Thousand Island:		
(Dia-Mel)	½-oz. pkg.	20
*(Weight Watchers)	1 T.	12
SALAMI:		
(Hormel):		
Cotto	1-oz. slice	65
Genoa, sliced	1-oz. slice	126
Hard, sliced	1-oz. slice	117
Party, sliced	1-oz. slice	94
(Oscar Mayer):		
For beer	.8-oz. slice	54
For beer, beef	.8-oz. slice	76
Cotto	.8-oz. slice	52
Cotto	.8-oz. slice	63
Hard	.3-oz. slice	33
(Swift) Genoa	1-oz. serving	114
(Vienna) beef	1-oz. serving	79
SALISBURY STEAK:		
Canned (Morton House)	6¼-oz. serving	160
Frozen:		
(Banquet):		
Buffet	2-lb. pkg.	1454
Man Pleaser	19-oz. dinner	873
(Green Giant) with gravy, oven bake	7-oz. serving	274

Food and Description	Measure or Quantity	Calories
(Morton) *Country Table*	12-oz. dinner	494
(Swanson):		
With gravy	10-oz. entree	440
Hungry Man	17-oz. dinner	870
3-course	16-oz. dinner	490
TV Brand	11½-oz. dinner	500
SALMON:		
Baked or broiled	6¾" x 2½" x 1"	264
Canned, regular pack:		
Keta (Bumble Bee) solids & liq.	½ cup	153
Pink or Humpback:		
(Bumble Bee) solids & liq.	½ cup	155
(Del Monte)	7¾-oz. can	277
Sockeye or Red or Blueback:		
(Bumble Bee) solids & liq.	½ cup	188
(Del Monte)	7¾-oz. can	330
Canned, dietetic (S&W) *Nutradiet*, low sodium	½ cup	188
SALMON, SMOKED (Vita):		
Lox, drained	4-oz. jar	136
Nova, drained	4-oz. can	221
SALT:		
(Morton) *Lite Salt*	1 tsp.	0
(Morton) Table	1 tsp.	0
Substitute:		
(Adolph's):		
Plain	1 tsp.	1
Seasoned	1 tsp.	6
(Morton) plain	1 tsp.	Tr.
Salt-It (Dia-Mel)	1 tsp.	0
SANDWICH SPREAD:		
(Hellmann's)	1 T.	64
(Oscar Mayer)	1-oz. serving	68
SANGRIA (Taylor)	3 fl. oz.	99
SARDINE, canned:		
Atlantic (Del Monte) with tomato sauce	7½-oz. can	330
Norwegian (Underwood):		
In mustard sauce	3¾-oz. can	195
In oil, drained	3¾-oz. can	233
In tomato sauce	3¾-oz. can	169
SAUCE:		
Regular pack:		
A-1	1 T.	12
Barbecue:		
Chris & Pitt's	1 T.	15

Food and Description	Measure or Quantity	Calories
(French's) regular or smoky	1 T.	25
(Gold's)	1 T.	16
Open Pit (General Foods) hickory smoke	1 T.	16
Cocktail:		
(Gold's)	1 T.	31
(Nalley's)	1-oz. serving	33
(Pfeiffer)	1-oz. serving	100
Escoffier Sauce Diable	1 T.	20
Escoffier Sauce Robert	1 T.	20
Famous Sauce	1 T.	69
Hot, *Frank's*	1 tsp.	1
Italian:		
(Carnation)	2 fl. oz.	43
(Ragu) red cooking	3½-oz. serving	45
Marinara (Ragu)	4-oz. serving	120
Mushroom (Nalley's)	1-oz. serving	17
Seafood (Bernstein's)	1 T.	16
Seafood cocktail (Del Monte)	1 T.	22
Soy:		
(Gold's)	1 T.	10
(Kikkoman)	1 T.	11
(La Choy)	1 T.	8
Spare rib (Gold's)	1 T.	51
Steak (Dawn Fresh) with mushrooms	1-oz. serving	9
Steak Supreme	1 T.	20
Sweet & sour:		
(Carnation)	2 fl. oz.	79
(La Choy)	1-oz. serving	51
Swiss steak (Carnation)	2-oz. serving	20
Taco:		
Old El Paso	1-oz. serving	11
(Ortega)	1 T.	22
Tartar:		
(Hellmann's)	1 T.	73
(Nalley's)	1 T.	89
Teriyaki (Kikkoman)	1 T.	14
V-8	1-oz. serving	25
White, medium	¼ cup	103
Worcestershire:		
(French's) regular or smoky	1 T.	10
(Gold's)	1 T.	42
SAUCE MIX:		
Regular:		
A la King (Durkee)	1-oz. pkg.	133

Food and Description	Measure or Quantity	Calories
*Cheese:		
(Durkee)	½ cup	168
(French's)	½ cup	160
Hollandaise:		
(Durkee)	1-oz. pkg.	173
*(French's)	1 T.	15
Sour cream:		
*(Durkee)	⅔ cup	214
*(French's)	2½ T.	60
*Stroganoff (French's)	⅛ cup	110
*Sweet & sour (Durkee)	1 cup	230
*Teriyaki (French's)	1 T.	17
*White (Durkee)	1 cup	238
*Dietetic (Weight Watchers) lemon butter	1 T.	8
SAUERKRAUT:		
(Claussen) drained	½ cup	16
(Del Monte) solids & liq.	1 cup	55
(Silver Floss):		
Regular, solids & liq.	½ cup	30
Bavarian Kraut, solids & liq.	½ cup	35
Krispy Kraut, solids & liq.	½ cup	25
SAUSAGE:		
Beef, *Cow-Boy Jo's*	⅝-oz. serving	81
Brown & serve (Swift) original	1 cooked link	77
SAUTERNE:		
(B&G)	3 fl. oz.	95
(Great Western)	3 fl. oz.	79
(Taylor)	3 fl. oz.	81
SCALLOP:		
Steamed	4-oz. serving	127
Frozen:		
(Mrs. Paul's):		
Breaded & fried	3½-oz. serving	201
With butter & cheese	7-oz. pkg.	260
(Van de Kamp's) country seasoned	3½-oz. serving	270
SCHAV SOUP (Gold's)	8-oz. serving	11
SCHNAPPS, PEPPERMINT (Mr. Boston)	1 fl. oz.	270
*SCOTCH BROTH SOUP (Campbell)	10-oz. serving	100
SCOTCH SOUR COCKTAIL, canned:		
(National Distillers) *Duet*, 12½% alcohol	2 fl. oz.	65
(Party Tyme) 12½% alcohol	2 fl. oz.	65

Food and Description	Measure or Quantity	Calories
SCREWDRIVER COCKTAIL:		
Canned:		
(Mr. Boston) 12½% alcohol	3 fl. oz.	111
(National Distillers) *Duet*, 12½% alcohol	3 fl. oz.	108
Mix, dry (Bar-Tender's)	1 serving	70
SEAFOOD PLATTER, frozen (Mrs. Paul's) breaded, fried	4½-oz. serving	254
SEGO DIET FOOD:		
Bars	1 bar	138
Canned, any flavor	10-fl.-oz. can	225
SERUTAN:		
Toasted granules	1 tsp.	6
Concentrated powder	1 tsp.	5
Fruit-flavored powder	1 tsp.	6
SESAME SEEDS (French's)	1 tsp.	9
SHAD, CREOLE	4-oz. serving	172
SHAKE 'N BAKE:		
Regular:		
Chicken	2.4-oz. serving	291
Chicken, barbecue style	3¾-oz. pkg.	377
Chicken, crispy country milk	2.3-oz. pkg.	321
Chicken, Italian flavor	2.3-oz. pkg.	294
Fish	2-oz. pkg.	234
Hamburger	2-oz. pkg.	169
Pork	2.4-oz. pkg.	255
Pork & ribs, barbecue style	2.9-oz. pkg.	305
Plus home-style gravy mix:		
Beef	3.2-oz. pkg.	304
Pork	3.7-oz. pkg.	327
SHERBET (Meadow Gold) orange	¼ pt.	120
SHERRY:		
Cocktail (Gold Seal)	3 fl. oz.	162
Cream:		
(Great Western)	3 fl. oz.	141
(Taylor)	3 fl. oz.	138
Dry:		
(Italian Swiss Colony) *Gold Medal*	3 fl. oz.	104
(Williams & Humbert)	3 fl. oz.	120
Dry Sack (Williams & Humbert)	3 fl. oz.	120
SHREDDED WHEAT:		
(Nabisco):		
Regular size	¾-oz. biscuit	90
Spoon Size	⅔ cup	110
(Quaker)	1 biscuit	52

Food and Description	Measure or Quantity	Calories
SHRIMP:		
Canned:		
(Bumble Bee) solids & liq.	4½-oz. can	138
(Icy Point) cocktail	4½-oz. can	148
Frozen (Mrs. Paul's) fried	3-oz. serving	198
SHRIMP CAKE, frozen		
(Mrs. Paul's) thins	2½-oz. cake	95
SHRIMP COCKTAIL:		
(Sau-Sea)	4-oz. jar	107
(Sea Snack)	4-oz. jar	110
SHRIMP DINNER, frozen		
(Van de Kamp's)	10-oz. dinner	270
SHRIMP PUFF (Durkee)	1 piece	44
SHRIMP SOUP:		
*(Campbell) cream of, made with milk	10-oz. serving	210
(Crosse & Blackwell)	6½-oz. serving	90
SHRIMP STICKS, frozen (Mrs. Paul's)	.8-oz. stick	48
SIRLOIN BURGER SOUP (Campbell) *Chunky*	10¾-oz. can	220
SLENDER (Carnation):		
Bar	1 bar	138
Dry	1 packet	110
Liquid	10-fl.-oz. can	225
SLIM JIM	1 piece	83
SLOPPY HOT DOG SEASONING MIX (French's)	1½-oz. pkg.	160
SLOPPY JOE:		
Canned:		
(Hormel) *Short Orders*	7½-oz. can	340
(Libby's):		
Beef	⅓ cup	119
Pork	⅓ cup	103
(Morton House) beef	5-oz. serving	240
(Nalley's)	8-oz. serving	348
Frozen:		
(Banquet) cooking bag	5-oz. bag	199
(Green Giant) with tomato sauce & beef, *Toast Topper*	5-oz. serving	154
SLOPPY JOE SEASONING MIX:		
*(Durkee):		
Regular flavor	1¼ cups	728
Pizza flavor	1¼ cups	746
(French's)	1½-oz. pkg.	128

Food and Description	Measure or Quantity	Calories
SMOKIE SAUSAGE:		
(Eckrich):		
Meat	1-oz. serving	105
Smok-Y-Links, skinless	.8-oz. link	85
(Hormel) smokies	1 link	80
(Oscar Mayer):		
Regular	1½-oz. link	137
Regular	4-oz. link	359
Beef	1½-oz. link	132
& cheese	1½-oz. link	142
(Vienna)	2½-oz. serving	196
SNO BALL (Hostess)	1 cake	140
SOAVE WINE (Antinori)	3 fl. oz.	84
SOFT DRINK:		
Sweetened:		
Aspen	6 fl. oz.	81
Bitter lemon:		
(Canada Dry)	6 fl. oz.	77
(Schweppes)	6 fl. oz.	84
Bubble Up	6 fl. oz.	73
Cherry:		
(Canada Dry) wild	6 fl. oz.	96
(Shasta) black	6 fl. oz.	86
Chocolate (Yoo-Hoo)	6 fl. oz.	108
Club (any brand)	6 fl. oz.	0
Coconut (Yoo-Hoo)	6 fl. oz.	89
Cola:		
Coca-Cola	6 fl. oz.	72
Jamaica (Canada Dry)	6 fl. oz.	79
Pepsi-Cola	6 fl. oz.	79
(Royal Crown)	6 fl. oz.	78
(Shasta)	6 fl. oz.	77
(Shasta) cherry	6 fl. oz.	74
Cream:		
(Canada Dry) vanilla	6 fl. oz.	96
(Schweppes) red	6 fl. oz.	86
(Shasta)	6 fl. oz.	81
Dr. Nehi (Royal Crown)	6 fl. oz.	73
Dr. Pepper	6 fl. oz.	75
Fruit Punch:		
(Nehi)	6 fl. oz.	91
(Shasta)	6 fl. oz.	84
Ginger ale:		
(Canada Dry)	6 fl. oz.	65
(Fanta)	6 fl. oz.	63
(Nehi)	6 fl. oz.	69
(Schweppes)	6 fl. oz.	66

Food and Description	Measure or Quantity	Calories
(Shasta)	6 fl. oz.	59
Ginger beer (Schweppes)	6 fl. oz.	72
Grape:		
(Canada Dry) concord	6 fl. oz.	96
(Fanta)	6 fl. oz.	86
(Hi-C)	6 fl. oz.	80
(Nehi)	6 fl. oz.	87
(Patio)	6 fl. oz.	96
(Schweppes)	6 fl. oz.	97
Grapefruit:		
(Cott)	6 fl. oz.	83
(Shasta)	6 fl. oz.	87
Hi-Spot (Canada Dry)	6 fl. oz.	74
Kick (Royal Crown)	6 fl. oz.	89
Lemonade (Hi-C)	6 fl. oz.	80
Lemon-lime (Shasta)	6 fl. oz.	70
Mello Yello	6 fl. oz.	87
Mountain Dew	6 fl. oz.	89
Mr. PiBB	6 fl. oz.	70
Orange:		
(Canada Dry) *Sunripe*	6 fl. oz.	90
(Fanta)	6 fl. oz.	88
(Hi-C)	6 fl. oz.	80
(Nehi)	6 fl. oz.	95
(Shasta)	6 fl. oz.	86
(Sunkist)	6 fl. oz.	96
Peach (Nehi)	6 fl. oz.	92
Quinine or Tonic Water:		
(Canada Dry)	6 fl. oz.	70
(Schweppes)	6 fl. oz.	66
Rondo (Schweppes)	6 fl. oz.	77
Root Beer:		
Barrelhead (Canada Dry)	6 fl. oz.	79
(Dad's)	6 fl. oz.	79
(Fanta)	6 fl. oz.	77
(Nehi)	6 fl. oz.	87
On Tap	6 fl. oz.	81
(Patio)	6 fl. oz.	83
Rooti (Canada Dry)	6 fl. oz.	79
(Shasta) draft	6 fl. oz.	75
Seven-Up	6 fl. oz.	72
Sprite	6 fl. oz.	71
Strawberry:		
(Canada Dry) California	6 fl. oz.	89
(Nehi)	6 fl. oz.	87
(Shasta)	6 fl. oz.	72
(Yoo-Hoo)	6 fl. oz.	95

Food and Description	Measure or Quantity	Calories
Tahatian Treat (Canada Dry)	6 fl. oz.	96
Teem	6 fl. oz.	61
Tom Collins or Collins Mix (Canada Dry)	6 fl. oz.	60
Upper 10 (Royal Crown)	6 fl. oz.	76
Vanilla:		
(Canada Dry) cream	6 fl. oz.	88
(Yoo-Hoo) shake	6 fl. oz.	93
Wink (Canada Dry)	6 fl. oz.	91
Dietetic or low calorie:		
Bubble Up	6 fl. oz.	1
Cherry:		
(Shasta)	6 fl. oz.	0
(Tab) black	6 fl. oz.	2
Chocolate (No-Cal) mint	6 fl. oz.	2
Cola:		
(Canada Dry)	6 fl. oz.	<1
Diet-Rite	6 fl. oz.	<1
(No-Cal)	6 fl. oz.	0
Pepsi, diet	6 fl. oz.	<1
Pepsi Light	6 fl. oz.	<1
RC (Royal Crown)	6 fl. oz.	<1
RC 100 (Royal Crown) caffeine-free	6 fl. oz.	<1
(Shasta) regular or cherry	6 fl. oz.	0
Tab	6 fl. oz.	<1
Dietetic or low calorie:		
Cream:		
(No-Cal)	6 fl. oz.	0
(Shasta)	6 fl. oz.	0
Dr. Pepper	6 fl. oz.	1
Fresca	6 fl. oz.	1
Ginger Ale:		
(Canada Dry)	6 fl. oz.	<1
(No-Cal)	6 fl. oz.	0
(Shasta)	6 fl. oz.	0
Tab	6 fl. oz.	2
Grape:		
(Shasta)	6 fl. oz.	0
Tab	6 fl. oz.	2
Grapefruit (Shasta)	6 fl. oz.	<1
Lemon (Shasta)	6 fl. oz.	0
Lemon-lime, *Tab*	6 fl. oz.	<1
Mr. PiBB	6 fl. oz.	<1
Orange:		
(No-Cal)	6 fl. oz.	0

Food and Description	Measure or Quantity	Calories
(Shasta)	6 fl. oz.	0
Tab	6 fl. oz.	<1
Quinine or Tonic (No-Cal)	6 fl. oz.	0
Raspberry (No-Cal) black	6 fl. oz.	2
Red Pop (No-Cal)	6 fl. oz.	0
Rondo (Schweppes)	6 fl. oz.	<1
Root Beer:		
Barrelhead (Canada Dry)	6 fl. oz.	<1
(Dad's)	6 fl. oz.	<1
(No-Cal)	6 fl. oz.	0
(Shasta) draft	6 fl. oz.	0
Tab	6 fl. oz.	<1
Seven-Up	6 fl. oz.	2
Shape-Up (No-Cal)	6 fl. oz.	0
Sprite	6 fl. oz.	2
Strawberry:		
(Shasta)	6 fl. oz.	0
Tab	6 fl. oz.	<2
Tab	6 fl. oz.	<1
TNT (No-Cal)	6 fl. oz.	0
SOLE, frozen:		
(Mrs. Paul's):		
Fillets, breaded & fried	4-oz. serving	225
Fillets, with lemon butter	4½-oz. serving	155
(Van de Kamp's) batter dipped, french fried	1 piece	140
(Weight Watchers)	16-oz. meal	245
SOUFFLÉ (Stouffer's) cheese	6-oz. serving	361
SOUP GREENS (Durkee)	2½-oz. jar	216
SOUTHERN COMFORT:		
86 proof	1 fl. oz.	84
100 proof	1 fl. oz.	96
SOYBEAN CURD or TOFU	2¾" x 1½" x 1" cake	86
SOYBEAN or NUT:		
Dry roasted (*Soy Ahoy; Soy Town*)	1 oz.	139
Oil roasted (*Soy Ahoy; Soy Town*) plain, barbecue or garlic flavored	1 oz.	152
SPAGHETTI, cooked:		
8-10 minutes, "al dente"	1 cup	216
14-20 minutes, tender	1 cup	155
SPAGHETTI DINNER, frozen (Swanson) TV Brand, in tomato sauce, with breaded veal	8½-oz. entree	290

Food and Description	Measure or Quantity	Calories
SPAGHETTI & MEATBALLS IN TOMATO SAUCE:		
Canned, regular pack:		
(Franco-American)	7⅜-oz. can	218
(Hormel) *Short Orders*	7½-oz. can	210
(Libby's)	7½-oz. serving	189
Canned, dietetic (Dia-Mel)	8-oz. can	200
Frozen:		
(Banquet)	8-oz. serving	282
(Green Giant)	9-oz. entree	269
(Morton)	11-oz. dinner	344
(Swanson) TV Brand	12½-oz. dinner	410
SPAGHETTI WITH MEAT SAUCE:		
Canned (Franco-American)	7½-oz. serving	220
Frozen:		
(Banquet)	8-oz. cooking bag	311
(Stouffer's)	14-oz. serving	442
SPAGHETTI Os **(Franco-American):**		
Tomato & cheese sauce	7⅜-oz. serving	160
Tomato sauce with little meatballs	7⅜-oz. serving	210
Tomato sauce with sliced franks	7⅜-oz. serving	210
SPAGHETTI SAUCE:		
Canned, regular pack:		
Clam (Ragu) chopped	5-oz. serving	110
Marinara:		
(Prince)	4-oz. serving	80
(Ragu)	5-oz. serving	120
Meat or meat flavored:		
(Prince)	½ cup	101
(Ragu)	5-oz. serving	115
(Ragu) extra thick & zesty	5-oz. serving	130
Meatless or plain:		
(Hain)	4-oz. serving	72
(Prince)	½ cup	90
(Ragu)	5-oz. serving	105
Mushroom:		
(Hain)	4-oz. serving	80
(Prince)	4-oz. serving	77
(Ragu)	5-oz. serving	105
(Ragu) extra thick & zesty	5-oz. serving	110
Pepperoni (Ragu)	5-oz. serving	120
Canned, dietetic pack (Featherweight)	⅔ cup	30
SPAGHETTI IN TOMATO SAUCE (Franco-American) with cheese	7⅜-oz. serving	170

Food and Description	*Measure or Quantity*	*Calories*
SPAM, luncheon meat (Hormel):		
Regular or smoke flavored	1-oz. serving	88
With cheese chunks	1-oz. serving	87
Deviled	1-oz. serving	78
SPECIAL K, cereal (Kellogg's)	1¼ cups	110
SPINACH:		
Fresh, whole leaves	½ cup	4
Boiled	½ cup	18
Canned, regular pack (Libby's) solids & liq.	½ cup	27
Canned, dietetic pack (Featherweight) solids & liq.	½ cup	35
Frozen:		
(Birds Eye):		
Chopped or leaf	⅓ of pkg.	23
Creamed	1/ of pkg.	57
(Green Giant):		
In butter sauce	⅓ of pkg.	42
Creamed	⅓ of pkg.	69
Souffle	½ of pkg.	109
(McKenzie)	⅓ of pkg.	27
(Seabrook Farms)	⅓ of pkg.	27
(Stouffer's) souffle	⅓ of pkg.	130
SQUASH, SUMMER:		
Yellow, boiled slices	½ of cup	13
Zucchini, boiled slices	½ cup	9
Canned (Del Monte) zucchini in tomato sauce	½ cup	37
Frozen:		
(McKenzie) Crookneck	⅓ of pkg.	22
(Seabrook Farms) Crookneck	⅓ of pkg.	22
(Seabrook Farms) Zucchini	3½-oz. serving	20
SQUASH, WINTER:		
Acorn, baked	½ cup	56
Hubbard, baked, mashed	½ cup	51
Frozen (Birds Eye)	⅓ of pkg.	50
****START***	½ cup	51
STEAK & GREEN PEPPERS, frozen (Swanson)	8½-oz. serving	200
STEAK & POTATO SOUP (Campbell) *Chunky*	19-oz. can	380
STOCK BASE (French's) beef or chicken	1 tsp.	8
***STOCKPOT SOUP** (Campbell) vegetable & beef	11-oz. serving	120
STRAWBERRY:		
Fresh, capped	½ cup	26

Food and Description	Measure or Quantity	Calories
Frozen (Birds Eye):		
Halves	⅓ of pkg.	196
Whole	¼ of pkg.	97
Whole, quick thaw	½ of pkg.	123
STRAWBERRY DRINK (Hi-C):		
Canned	6 fl. oz.	89
*Mix	6 fl. oz.	68
STRAWBERRY ICE CREAM:		
(Meadow Gold)	¼ pt.	140
(Swift)	½ cup	124
STRAWBERRY PRESERVE OR JAM:		
Sweetened (Smucker's)	1 T.	53
Dietetic or low calorie:		
(Diet Delight)	1 T.	13
(Featherweight)	1 T.	16
(Featherweight) artificially sweetened	1 T.	6
(Slenderella) imitation	1 T.	24
(S&W) *Nutradiet*	1 T.	12
STUFFING MIX:		
*Chicken, *Stove Top*	½ cup	170
*Cornbread, *Stove Top*	½ cup	170
*Pork, *Stove Top*	½ cup	170
White bread, *Mrs. Cubbison's*	1 oz.	101
STURGEON, smoked	4-oz. serving	169
SUCCOTASH:		
Canned:		
(Libby's) cream style	½ cup	111
(Libby's) whole kernel	½ cup	82
(Stokely-Van Camp)	½ cup	85
Frozen (Birds Eye)	⅓ of pkg.	80
SUGAR:		
Brown	1 T.	48
Confectioners'	1 T.	30
Granulated	1 T.	46
Maple	1¾" x 1¼" x ½" piece	104
SUGAR CORN POPS, cereal	1 cup	110
SUGAR CRISP, cereal	⅞ cup	113
SUGAR SMACKS, cereal (Kellogg's)	¾ cup	110
SUGAR SUBSTITUTE:		
(Featherweight)	3 drops	0
Sprinkle Sweet (Pillsbury)	⅛ tsp.	2
Sugar-Like (Dia-Mel)	1 packet	3
Sweet'n-it (Dia-Mel) liquid	5 drops	0

Food and Description	Measure or Quantity	Calories
*SUKIYAKI DINNER, frozen (Chun King) stir fry	⅛ of pkg.	100
SUNDAE, canned, *Swiss Miss*:		
Chocolate	4½ oz.	190
Vanilla	4½ oz.	180
SUNFLOWER SEED:		
In hulls	1 oz.	86
Hulled (Planters)	1 oz.	164
Dry roasted (Planters)	1 oz.	160
SUZY Q (Hostess):		
Banana	1 cake	244
Chocolate	1 cake	240
SWEETBREADS, calf, braised	4-oz. serving	191
SWEET POTATO:		
Baked, peeled	5" x 1" potato	155
Canned, heavy syrup	4-oz. serving	129
Frozen:		
(Green Giant) glazed	⅓ of pkg.	120
(Mrs. Paul's) candied, with apple	4-oz. serving	162
*SWEET & SOUR DINNER, frozen (Chun King) stir fry	⅛ of pkg.	140
SWEET & SOUR PORK (Chun King)	½ of 12-oz. pouch	200
SWEET & SOUR ORIENTAL, canned (La Choy):		
—Chicken	8½-oz. serving	340
Pork	8½-oz. serving	361
SWISS STEAK, frozen (Swanson)	10-oz. dinner	350
SWORDFISH, broiled	3" x 3" x ½" steak	218
SYRUP (See also TOPPING):		
Regular:		
Apricot (Smucker's)	1 T.	50
Blackberry (Smucker's)	1 T.	50
Chocolate or chocolate-flavored:		
Bosco	1 T.	55
Corn, *Karo*, dark or light	1 T.	58
Maple, *Karo*, imitation	1 T.	57
Pancake or waffle:		
Aunt Jemima	¼ cup	212
Golden Griddle	1 T.	54
Karo	1 T.	58
Log Cabin, regular	1 T.	52
Mrs. Butterworth's	1 T.	55
Strawberry (Smucker's)	1 T.	50
Dietetic or low calorie:		
Blueberry (Featherweight)	1 T.	14

Food and Description	Measure or Quantity	Calories
Chocolate-flavored (Featherweight)	1 T.	30
Coffee (No-Cal)	1 T.	6
Cola (No-Cal)	1 T.	0
Maple (S&W) *Nutradiet*	1 T.	12
Pancake or waffle:		
(Diet Delight)	1 T.	14
(Featherweight)	1 T.	12
(Tillie Lewis) *Tasti-Diet*	1 T.	13

T

Food and Description	Measure or Quantity	Calories
TABASCO	½ tsp.	<1
TACO:		
*(Ortega)	1 taco	220
*Mix (Durkee)	½ cup	321
Shell (Ortega)	1 shell	50
TAMALE:		
Canned:		
(Hormel) beef, *Short Orders*	7½-oz. can	270
(Nalley's) beef	8-oz. serving	268
(Nalley's) chicken	8-oz. serving	209
Old El Paso, with chili gravy	1 tamale	116
Frozen (Hormel) beef	1 tamale	130
TAMALE PIE (Nalley's)	4-oz. serving	113
***TANG**, grape or orange	½ cup	64
TANGERINE or MANDARIN ORANGE:		
Fresh (Sunkist)	1 large tangerine	39
Canned, regular pack (Del Monte) solids & liq.	5½-oz. serving	106
Canned, dietetic:		
(Featherweight) water pack	½ cup	35
(S&W) *Nutradiet*	½ cup	28
TANGERINE DRINK, canned (Hi-C)	6 fl. oz.	90
***TANGERINE JUICE**, frozen (Minute Maid)	6 fl. oz.	85
TARRAGON (French's)	1 tsp.	5
***TASTEEOS**, cereal (Ralston Purina)	1¼ cups	110
TEA:		
(Lipton)	1 teabag	0
(Tender Leaf)	1 rounded tsp.	1
Canned (Lipton) lemon flavor	12-fl.-oz. can	130
***TEAM**, cereal	1 cup	110

Food and Description	Measure or Quantity	Calories
TEA MIX, iced:		
*(Lipton) lemon flavored	1 cup	60
*Nestea, lemon-flavored	8 fl. oz.	20
TEMPTYS (Tastykake) chocolate cream	2-oz. pkg.	197
TERIYAKI, frozen (Stouffer's) beef, with rice & vegetables	10-oz. serving	367
TEQUILA SUNRISE COCKTAIL, canned (Mr. Boston) 12½% alcohol	3 fl. oz.	120
***TEXTURED VEGETABLE PROTEIN,** Morningstar Farms:*		
Breakfast link	1 link	62
Breakfast patties	1 patty	109
Breakfast strips	1 strip	34
Grillers	1 pattie	189
THURINGER:		
(Hormel):		
Buffet	1-oz. serving	95
Old Smokehouse	1-oz. serving	100
(Oscar Mayer) beef	.8-oz. slice	72
TIGER TAILS (Hostess)	1 piece	222
TOASTER CAKE OR PASTRY:		
Flavor-Kist (Schulze and Burch):		
Regular:		
All flavors except brown sugar cinnamon	1 pastry	190
Brown sugar cinnamon	1 pastry	200
Frosted:		
Apple, blueberry, cherry or strawberry	1 pastry	190
Brown sugar cinnamon	1 pastry	200
Fudge	1 pastry	195
Pop-Tarts (Kellogg's)		
Regular	1 pastry	210
Frosted:		
All flavors except chocolate fudge or chocolate-vanilla creme	1 pastry	210
Chocolate fudge or chocolate-vanilla creme	1 pastry	200
Toastettes (Nabisco)	1 pastry	190
Toast-R-Cake (Thomas')		
Blueberry	1 piece	110
Bran	1 piece	112
Corn	1 piece	116
TOASTY O's, cereal	1¼ cups	113

Food and Description	Measure or Quantity	Calories
TOMATO:		
Cherry, whole	4 pieces	14
Regular, whole	1 med. tomato	33
Canned, regular pack:		
(Contadina) sliced	4-oz. serving	35
(Stokely-Van Camp) stewed	½ cup	35
(Van Camp) whole	½ cup	25
Canned, dietetic pack:		
(Featherweight)	½ cup	20
(S&W) *Nutradiet*, whole	½ cup	25
(Tillie Lewis) *Tasti-Diet*	½ cup	25
TOMATO JUICE:		
Canned, regular pack:		
(Campbell)	6-fl.-oz. can	40
(Del Monte)	6-fl.-oz. can	36
Musselman's	6 fl. oz.	30
Canned, dietetic pack:		
(Featherweight)	6 fl. oz.	35
(S&W) *Nutradiet*	6 fl. oz.	35
TOMATO JUICE COCKTAIL:		
(Ocean Spray) *Firehouse Jubilee*	6 fl. oz.	44
Snap-E-Tom	6 fl. oz.	40
TOMATO PASTE, canned:		
Regular pack:		
(Del Monte)	6-oz. can	164
(Hunt's)	6-oz. can	140
Dietetic (Featherweight) low sodium	6-oz. can	150
TOMATO & PEPPER, HOT CHILI (Ortega) Jalapeno	1-oz. serving	7
TOMATO, PICKLED (Claussen) green	1 piece	6
TOMATO PUREE, canned:		
Regular (Contadina) heavy	1 cup	110
Dietetic (Featherweight)	1 cup	90
TOMATO SAUCE, canned:		
(Contadina)	1 cup	87
(Del Monte):		
Regular	1 cup	85
With tomato tidbits	1 cup	130
(Hunt's) with cheese	4-oz. serving	70
TOMATO SOUP, canned:		
Regular pack (Campbell):		
*Made with milk	10-oz. serving	210
*Made with water	10-oz. serving	110
*Bisque	11-oz. serving	160

Food and Description	Measure or Quantity	Calories
*Rice, old fashioned	11-oz. serving	150
Soup For One, Royale	7¾-oz. can	180
Dietetic pack:		
(Campbell) low sodium	7¼-oz. can	130
*(Dia-Mel)	8-oz. serving	50
TOMATO SOUP MIX:		
*(Lipton) Cup-a-Soup	6 fl. oz.	70
*(Nestlé) Souptime	6 fl. oz.	70
TONGUE, beef, braised	4-oz. serving	277
TOPPING:		
Regular:		
Butterscotch (Smucker's)	1 T.	70
Caramel (Smucker's)	1 T.	70
Chocolate fudge (Hershey's)	1 T.	49
Peanut butter caramel (Smucker's)	1 T.	75
Pecans in syrup (Smucker's)	1 T.	65
Pineapple (Smucker's)	1 T.	65
Dietetic, chocolate (Diet Delight)	1 T.	16
TOPPING, WHIPPED:		
Regular:		
Cool Whip (Birds Eye)	1 T.	19
Lucky Whip, aerosol	1 T.	12
Richwhip	1 T.	20
Whip Topping (Rich's)	¼ oz.	20
Dietetic (Featherweight)	1 T.	3
*Mix (Dream Whip)	1 T.	10
TOP RAMEN, beef (Nissin Foods)	3-oz. serving	390
TORTILLA (Amigos)	6" x ⅛" tortilla	111
TOSTADA SHELL (Ortega)	1 shell	50
TOTAL, cereal	1 cup	110
TRAMINER WINE (Inglenook)	3 fl. oz.	60
TRIPE, canned (Libby's)	6-oz. serving	290
TRIPLE SEC LIQUEUR (Mr. Boston)	1 fl. oz.	79
TRIX, cereal (General Mills)	1 cup	110
TROUT, frozen, dressed (1000 Springs)	5-oz. trout	164
TUNA:		
Canned in oil:		
(Breast O'Chicken) solids & liq.	6½-oz. can	427
(Bumble Bee):		
Chunk, light, drained	6½-oz. can	309
Solids, white, drained	7-oz. can	333
(Carnation) solids & liq.	6½-oz. can	427
(Chicken of the Sea) chunk, light, solids & liq.	6½-oz. can	405

Food and Description	Measure or Quantity	Calories
(Star Kist) solids, white, solids & liq.	7-oz. serving	503
Canned in water:		
(Breast O' Chicken)	6½-oz. can	211
(Bumble Bee):		
Chunk, light, solids & liq.	6½-oz. can	234
Solid, white, solids & liq.	7-oz. can	251
(Star Kist) light	7-oz. can	220
(Chicken of the Sea) white	7-oz. can	240
*TUNA HELPER (General Mills):		
Cheese sauce & country dumplings	⅕ of pkg.	230
Creamy noodle	⅕ of pkg.	280
TUNA NOODLE CASSEROLE, frozen (Stouffer's)	5¾-oz. serving	193
TUNA & PEAS, frozen (Green Giant) creamed	5-oz. serving	136
TUNA PIE, frozen:		
(Banquet)	8-oz. pie	479
(Morton)	8-oz. pie	373
TUNA SALAD:		
Home recipe	4-oz. serving	193
Canned (Carnation)	1½-oz. serving	81
TURBOT MEAL, frozen (Weight Watchers):		
Regular	8-oz. meal	316
Stuffed	16-oz. meal	420
TURKEY:		
Canned:		
(Hormel) chunk	6¾-oz. serving	223
(Swanson) chunk	2½-oz. serving	120
Packaged:		
(Eckrich) sliced	1-oz. serving	47
(Hormel) breast	.8-oz. slice	29
(Oscar Mayer) breast	¾-oz. slice	21
Roasted:		
Flesh & skin	4-oz. serving	253
Dark meat	2½" x 1⅝" x ¼" slice	43
Light meat	4" x 2" x ¼" slice	75
TURKEY DINNER OR ENTREE, frozen		
(Banquet):		
Regular	11-oz. dinner	293
Man Pleaser	19-oz. dinner	620
(Morton):		
King Size	19-oz. dinner	582
Sliced, *Country Table*	15-oz. dinner	580

Food and Description	Measure or Quantity	Calories
(Swanson):		
With gravy & dressing	9-oz. entree	310
Hungry Man	19-oz. dinner	750
(Weight Watchers) sliced	16-oz. meal	350
TURKEY PIE, frozen:		
(Banquet)	8-oz. pie	415
(Morton)	8-oz. pie	334
(Stouffer's)	10-oz. pie	451
(Swanson):		
Regular	8-oz. pie	460
Hungry Man	1-lb. pie	800
TURKEY SOUP (Campbell):		
Regular:		
Chunky	18½-oz. can	280
*Condensed, noodle	10-oz. serving	80
Dietetic, low sodium	7¼-oz. can	60
TURKEY TETRAZINI, frozen		
(Stouffer's)	6-oz. serving	248
TUMERIC (French's)	1 tsp.	7
TURNOVER:		
Frozen (Pepperidge Farm):		
Apple	1 turnover	310
Blueberry or peach	1 turnover	320
Cherry or raspberry	1 turnover	340
Refrigerated (Pillsbury):		
Apple or blueberry	1 turnover	170
Cherry	1 turnover	180
TWINKIE (Hostess):		
Regular	1 cake	147
Devil's food	1 cake	150

V

VALPOLICELLA WINE		
(Antinori)	3 fl. oz.	84
VANDERMINT, liqueur	1 fl. oz.	90
VANILLA EXTRACT		
(Virginia Dare)	1 tsp.	10
VANILLA ICE CREAM:		
(Meadow Gold)	¼ pt.	140
(Swift)	½ cup	127
VEAL, broiled, medium cooked:		
Loin chop	4 oz.	265
Rib, roasted	4 oz.	305
Steak or cutlet, lean & fat	4 oz.	245

Food and Description	Measure or Quantity	Calories
VEAL DINNER, frozen:		
(Banquet) parmigiana	11-oz. dinner	421
(Green Giant) parmigiana	7-oz. serving	310
(Morton) parmigiana	11-oz. dinner	272
(Swanson):		
Hungry Man, parmigiana	20½-oz. dinner	990
TV Brand, parmigiana	12¼-oz. dinner	510
VEAL STEAK, frozen (Hormel):		
Regular	4-oz. serving	131
Breaded	4-oz. serving	242
VEGETABLE JUICE COCKTAIL:		
Regular, V-8	6 fl. oz.	39
Dietetic:		
(S&W) *Nutradiet,* low sodium	6 fl. oz.	35
V-8, low sodium	6 fl. oz.	40
VEGETABLES, MIXED:		
Canned, regular pack:		
(Chun King) chow mein, solids & liq.	4-oz. serving	20
(Del Monte) drained	½ cup	41
(La Choy):		
Chinese	1 cup	24
Chop Suey	1 cup	36
(Libby's) solids & liq.	½ cup	40
(Stokely-Van Camp) solids & liq.	½ cup	40
(Veg-All)	½ cup	39
Canned, dietetic pack (Featherweight)	½ cup	40
Frozen:		
(Birds Eye):		
Americana Recipe:		
New England style	⅓ of pkg.	69
New Orleans style	⅓ of pkg.	69
Pennsylvania Dutch style	⅓ of pkg.	44
San Francisco style	⅓ of pkg.	42
Wisconsin style	⅓ of pkg.	44
International Style:		
Bavarian style	⅓ of pkg.	63
Chinese style	⅓ of pkg.	50
Italian style	⅓ of pkg.	50
Japanese style	⅓ of pkg.	42
Stir Fry:		
Chinese style	⅓ of pkg.	35
Mandarin style	⅓ of pkg.	30
(Green Giant):		
Chinese style	½ cup	65

Food and Description	Measure or Quantity	Calories
Hawaiian style	½ cup	100
Mixed	½ cup	45
(Kounty Kist)	½ cup	45
(La Choy):		
Chinese	5-oz. serving	36
Japanese	5-oz. serving	36
(Ore-Ida) stew vegetables	⅛ of 24-oz. pkg.	60
VEGETABLE SOUP, canned:		
Regular pack (Campbell):		
Chunky:	10¾-oz. can	140
*Condensed:		
Regular	10-oz. serving	100
Beef	10-oz. serving	90
Old fashioned	10-oz. serving	90
Soup For One, beef, burly	7¾-oz. can	150
Soup For One, old world	7¾-oz. can	120
Vegetarian	10-oz. serving	90
Dietetic:		
(Campbell) low sodium	7¼-oz. can	90
*(Dia-Mel)	8-oz. serving	60
VEGETABLE SOUP MIX:		
*(Lipton):		
Alphabet, *Cup-A-Soup*	1 pkg.	40
Beef	1 cup	60
Italian vegetable	1 cup	100
*(Nestlé) *Souptime,* cream of	1 envelope	80
VEGETABLE STEW, canned, *Dinty Moore*	7½-oz. serving	163
"VEGETARIAN FOODS":		
Canned or dry:		
Chicken, fried (Loma Linda) with gravy	1½-oz. piece	109
Chili (Worthington)	¼ can (5-oz. serving)	190
Choplet (Worthington)	1 choplet	50
Dinner cuts (Loma Linda) drained	1 cut	54
Dinner cuts (Loma Linda) drained, no salt added	1 cut	44
Franks, big (Loma Linda)	1.9-oz. frank	100
Franks, sizzle (Loma Linda)	2.2-oz. frank	167
FriChik (Worthington)	1 piece	95
Granburger (Worthington)	6 T.	130
Linketts (Loma Linda) drained	1.3-oz. link	74
Little links (Loma Linda) drained	.8-oz. link	45
Non-meatballs (Worthington)	1 meatball	165
Nuteena (Loma Linda)	½" slice	165

Food and Description	Measure or Quantity	Calories
Proteena (Loma Linda)	½" slice	144
Redi-burger (Loma Linda)	½" slice	132
Sandwich spread:		
(Loma Linda)	1 T.	24
(Worthington)	2½ oz.	120
Savorex (Loma Linda)	1 T.	32
Soyagen, all purpose powder (Loma Linda)	1 T.	48
Soyalac (Loma Linda):		
I-soyalac	1 cup	177
Concentrate, liquid	1 cup	351
Ready to use	1 cup	166
Soyameat (Worthington):		
Sliced beef	1 slice	55
Diced chicken	¼ cup	120
Sliced chicken	1 slice	65
Salisbury steak	1 slice	160
Soyamel, any kind (Worthington)	1 oz.	145
Stew pack (Loma Linda) drained	1 piece	7
Super links (Worthington)	1 link	120
Swiss steak with gravy (Loma Linda)	1 steak	138
Tender bits (Loma Linda) drained	1 piece	23
Vege-burger (Loma Linda)	½ cup	116
Vege-burger (Loma Linda) no salt added	½ cup	119
Vegelona (Loma Linda)	½" slice	102
Vega-Links (Worthington)	1 link	70
Vita-burger (Loma Linda)	1 T.	23
Wheat protein	4 oz.	124
Worthington 209	1 slice	75
Frozen:		
Beef-like slices (Worthington)	1 slice	60
Beef pie (Worthington)	1 pie	470
Bologna (Loma Linda)	1 oz.	77
Chicken (Loma Linda)	1 slice	57
Chicken, fried (Loma Linda)	2-oz. serving	188
Chicken pie (Worthington)	1 pie	450
Chic-Ketts (Worthington)	½ cup	180
Corned beef, loaf, or sliced (Worthington)	2½ oz.	190
FriPats (Worthington)	1 pat	180
Meatballs (Loma Linda)	1 meatball	46
Prosage (Worthington)	1 link	60

Food and Description	Measure or Quantity	Calories
Roast Beef (Loma Linda)	1 oz.	65
Sausage, breakfast (Loma Linda)	⅛" slice	72
Smoked beef, roll (Worthington)	2½ oz.	170
Stripples (Worthington)	1 slice	25
Turkey (Loma Linda)	1 oz.	61
Wham, roll (Worthington)	2½ oz.	140
VERMOUTH:		
Dry & extra dry (Lejon; Noilly Pratt)	1 fl. oz.	33
Sweet (Lejon; Taylor)	1 fl. oz.	45
VICHYSSOISE SOUP (Crosse & Blackwell) cream of	6½-oz. serving	70
VIENNA SAUSAGE:		
(Hormel):		
Regular	1 sausage	53
Chicken	1-oz. serving	60
(Libby's)	.7-oz. sausage	50
VINEGAR	1 T.	2

W

Food and Description	Measure or Quantity	Calories
WAFFELOS, cereal (Ralston Purina)	1 cup	110
WAFFLE, frozen:		
(Aunt Jemima) jumbo	1 waffle	86
(Downyflake) jumbo	1 waffle	130
(Eggo):		
Blueberry or strawberry	1 waffle	130
Home style	1 waffle	120
WALLBANGER COCKTAIL, canned (Mr. Boston) 12½% alcohol	3 fl. oz.	102
WALNUT, English or Persian (Diamond A)	1 cup	679
WALNUT FLAVORING, BLACK (Durkee) imitation	1 tsp.	4
WATER CHESTNUT, canned:		
(Chun King) solids & liq.	8½-oz. can	140
(La Choy) drained	8-oz. can	65
WATERCRESS, trimmed	½ cup	3
WATERMELON:		
Wedge	4" x 8" wedge	111
Diced	½ cup	21

Food and Description	Measure or Quantity	Calories
WIENER WRAP, refrigerated (Pillsbury)	1 piece	60
WELSH RAREBIT:		
Home recipe	1 cup	415
Frozen:		
(Green Giant)	5-oz. serving	219
(Stouffer's)	5-oz. serving	359
WESTERN DINNER, frozen:		
(Banquet)	11-oz. dinner	417
(Morton) *Round-Up*	11.8-oz. dinner	426
(Swanson):		
Hungry Man	17¾-oz. dinner	840
TV Brand	11¾-oz. dinner	440
WHEAT CHEX, cereal	⅔ cup	100
WHEATENA, cereal	¼ cup	112
WHEAT FLAKES CEREAL:		
(Breakfast Best)	1 cup	141
(Van Brode)	¾ cup	106
WHEAT GERM CEREAL:		
(Kellogg's) all flavors	¼ cup	110
(Kretschmer) all flavors	¼ cup	110
WHEATIES, cereal	1 cup	110
WHEAT & RAISIN CHEX, cereal (Ralston Purina)	¾ cup	120
WHISKEY SOUR COCKTAIL, canned:		
(Hiram Walker)	3 fl. oz.	177
(Mr. Boston) 12½% alcohol	3 fl. oz.	120
WHITEFISH, LAKE:		
Baked, stuffed	4 oz.	244
Smoked	4 oz.	176
WILD BERRY DRINK, canned (Hi-C)	6 fl. oz.	88
WINE, COOKING (Regina):		
Burgundy or sauterne	¼ cup	2
Sherry	¼ cup	20
WON TON SOUP:		
Canned (Mow Sang)	10-oz. can	134
*Frozen (La Choy)	1 cup	92

Food and Description	Measure or Quantity	Calories

Y

YEAST, BAKER'S (Fleischmann's):

Dry, active	¼ oz.	20
Fresh & household, active	.6-oz. cake	15

YOGURT:
Regular:
 Plain:

(Dannon)	8-oz. container	150
Viva	8-oz. container	180
Yoplait	6-oz. container	130
Apple, Yoplait	6-oz. container	190
Apple crisp (New Country)	8-oz. container	240
Apricot (Dannon)	8-oz. container	260
Banana (Dannon)	8-oz. container	260
Blueberry:		
(Dannon)	8-oz. container	260
(Sweet'N Low)	8-oz. container	150
Yoplait	6-oz. container	190
Blueberry ripple (New Country)	8-oz. container	240
Boysenberry (Dannon)	8-oz. container	260
Cherry:		
(Dannon)	8-oz. container	260
(Sweet'N Low)	8-oz. container	150
Yoplait	6-oz. container	190
Cherry supreme (New Country)	8-oz. container	240
Coffee (Dannon)	8-oz. container	200
Dutch apple (Dannon)	8-oz. container	260
Flavored (Alta-Dena):		
Maya	1 container	280
Naja	1 container	250
French vanilla ripple (New Country)	8-oz. container	240
Fruit crunch (New Country)	8-oz. container	240
Hawaiian salad (New Country)	8-oz. container	250
Honey (Dannon)	8-oz. container	260
Honey'n Berries (New Country)	8-oz. container	240
Lemon:		
(Dannon)	8-oz. container	200
(Sweet'N Low)	8-oz. container	150
Yoplait	6-oz. container	190
Lemon ripple (New Country)	8-oz. container	240

Food and Description	Measure or Quantity	Calories
Orange, *Yoplait*	6-oz. container	190
Orange supreme (New Country)	8-oz. container	240
Peach:		
(Dannon)	8-oz. container	260
(Sweet'N Low)	8-oz. container	150
Peaches'n Cream (New Country)	8-oz. container	240
Pineapple-orange (Dannon)	8-oz. container	260
Raspberry:		
(Dannon) red	8-oz. container	260
(Sweet'N Low)	8-oz. container	150
Yoplait	6-oz. container	190
Raspberry ripple (New Country)	8-oz. container	240
Strawberry:		
(Dannon)	8-oz. container	260
(Sweet'N Low)	8-oz. container	150
Viva, Swiss style	8-oz. container	250
Yoplait	6-oz. container	190
Strawberry supreme (New Country)	8-oz. container	240
Vanilla (Dannon)	8-oz. container	200
Frozen (Dannon):		
Banana:		
Danny-Yo	3½-oz. serving	110
Danny-in-a-Cup	8-oz. cup	210
Blueberry, *Danny Parfait*	4-oz. serving	160
Boysenberry:		
Danny-On-A-Stick, carob coated	2½-fl.-oz. bar	135
Danny-Yo	3½-oz. serving	110
Cherry, *Danny-in-a-Cup*	1 cup	210
Chocolate, *Danny-Yo*	3½-oz. serving	110
Lemon, *Danny-in-a-Cup*	8-oz. cup	180
Peach:		
Danny-in-a-Cup	8-oz. cup	210
Danny Parfait	4-oz. serving	160
Pina Colada:		
Danny-in-a-Cup	8-oz. cup	210
Danny-On-A-Stick	2½-fl.-oz. bar	65
Pineapple-orange, *Danny Parfait*	4-oz. serving	160
Raspberry, red:		
Danny-On-A-Stick, chocolate coated	2½-fl.-oz. bar	135
Danny-in-a-Cup	8-oz. container	210

Food and Description	Measure or Quantity	Calories
Danny Parfait	4-oz. serving	160
Strawberry:		
Danny-in-a-Cup	8-oz. cup	210
Danny Flip, with strawberry topping	5-fl.-oz. serving	175
Danny Parfait	4-oz. serving	160
Danny-On-A-Stick	2½-fl.-oz. bar	65
Danny-On-A-Stick, chocolate coated	2½-fl.-oz. bar	135
Danny-Yo	3½-oz. serving	110
Vanilla:		
Danny-in-a-Cup	8-oz. cup	180
Danny Flip, with red raspberry topping	5 fl. oz.	175
Danny-On-A-Stick	2½-fl.-oz. bar	65
Danny-On-A-Stick, carob coated	2½-fl.-oz. bar	135
Danny-Yo	3½-oz. serving	110
Vanilla-strawberry, Danny Sampler	3-fl.-oz. serving	70

Z

ZINFANDEL WINE:		
(Inglenook) Vintage	3 fl. oz.	59
(Italian Swiss Colony)	3 fl. oz.	61
ZITI, frozen (Ronzoni)	4½-oz. serving	130
ZWIEBACK (Nabisco)	1 piece	30